ABC OF DERMATOLOGY

Fourth Edition

ABC OF
DERMATOLOGY

Fourth Edition

PAUL K BUXTON

Consultant Dermatologist
Royal Infirmary, Edinburgh

First published by the BMJ Publishing Group Ltd in 1988
Second edition 1993
Third edition 1998
Hot Climates edition 1999
Fourth edition 2003
Second impression 2004
Third impression 2005
Fourth impression 2005

BMJ Publishing Group Ltd, BMA House, Tavistock Square,
London WC1H 9JR

British Library Cataloguing in Publication Data
A catalogue record for this book is available from the British Library

ISBN 0-7279-1696-3

Typeset by Newgen Imaging Systems (P) Ltd., Chennai, India
Printed and bound in Spain by Graphycems
Cover picture is a light micrograph of a vertical section through a human
skull showing several hair follicles. With permission of
Dr Clive Kocher/Science Photo Library

Contents

Contributors

R Balfour
General Practitioner, Edinburgh

R StC Barnetson
Professor of Dermatology, Department of Dermatology,
Prince Albert Hospital, Camperdown, Australia

E Crawford
General Practitioner, Edinburgh

DJ Gawkrodger
Consultant Dermatologist, Royal Hallamshire Hospital, Sheffield

DWS Harris
Consultant Dermatologist, Whittington Hospital, London

RJ Hay
Dean, Faculty of Medicine and Health Sciences
and Professor of Dermatology, Queens University, Belfast

D Kemmett
Consultant Dermatologist, Lothian University NHS Trust,
Edinburgh

B Leppard
Professor, Regional Dermatology Training Centre, Moshi,
Tanzania

JA Savin
Consultant Dermatologist, Lothian University NHS Trust,
Edinburgh

MA Waugh
Consultant in Genitourinary Medicine, Leeds Teaching
Hospitals NHS Trust, Leeds

AL Wright
Consultant Dermatologist, Bradford Royal Infirmary

Acknowledgements

Professor R StC Barnetson, University of Sydney, Australia, wrote the original chapter on the sun and the skin, which is included in this edition. Professor Barbara Leppard, Regional Dermatology Training Centre, Moshi, Tanzania, has contributed a chapter on tropical dermatology with her own illustrations and some from Professor Barnetson. Professor R Hay, St Johns Institute of Dermatology, UMDS, Guy's Hospital, London, extensively revised the section on bacterial and fungal infections and provided some illustrations. Dr JA Savin, Lothian University NHS Trust, Edinburgh, rewrote the section on genetics and skin disease. Dr MA Waugh, consultant in GU medicine, The Leeds Teaching Hospitals NHS Trust, provided material and illustrations on AIDS. Dr Robin Balfour and Dr Ewan Crawford, general practitioners in Edinburgh, provided contributions on dermatology in general practice.

Material from contributors to earlier editions has been retained, particularly that supplied by Dr DJ Gawkrodger, consultant dermatologist, Royal Hallamshire Hospital, Sheffield (autoimmunity), Dr DWS Harris, consultant dermatologist, Whittington Hospital, London (practical procedures), Dr D Kemmett, consultant dermatologist, Lothian University NHS Trust, Edinburgh (diseases of hair and scalp), Dr AL Wright, consultant dermatologist, Bradford Royal Infirmary (diseases of nails).

The illustrations come from the Fife hospitals, the Royal Infirmary Edinburgh and the author's own collection. Some specific illustrations have been donated by Dr JA Savin (flea bites on the ankle); Dr Peter Ball (rubella); Professor CV Ruckley (varicose veins); Dr GB Colver (spider naevus); Dr MA Waugh and Dr M Jones (AIDS); Dr PMW Copemen (dermatoses in black skin). Miss Julie Close made the diagrams of the nail and types of immune response. The illustrations for dermatology in general practice were produced by Sister Sheila Robertson, Dermatology Liaison Nurse in Fife and Julie Close. The text of the third edition, on which this one is based, was typed by Mrs Mary Henderson. I would also like to thank Pat Croucher, who proofread the third edition, for copy-editing the script for this edition with perception and patience. Sally Carter and the editorial staff at BMJ Books gave great help and support.

Finally thanks are due to all the hospital staff—and particularly the patients—without whom dermatology could not be practised at all.

Preface

The remit for the first edition of the *ABC of Dermatology* in 1987 was that it should concentrate on common conditions and give down to earth advice. The ABC format proved well suited for this and there has been a steady demand for the book since then. In this edition the same approach is maintained while taking into account advances in diagnosis and treatment. Research in genetics and immunology is providing ever-increasing insights into the mechanisms that underlie clinical changes, and has led to more accurate diagnosis and more rational treatment. Specialised techniques that may not be relevant to common conditions can be of the greatest importance to an individual patient with a rare disease. In epidermolysis bullosa, for example, the ability to differentiate accurately between the different types with electronmicroscopy and immunohistochemistry is of considerable significance. Generally research increases our understanding of *how* diseases arise, but we have to admit to ourselves and our patients that *why* they occur remains as elusive as ever.

In recent years the management of inflammatory skin conditions has become both more effective and less demanding for the patient. In addition there is greater recognition of the impact of skin diseases on the patient's life. Major advances in treatment include more effective and safer phototherapy and the use of immunosuppressive drugs that enable inflammatory dermatoses to be managed without the need to attend for dressings or admission to hospital. This is just as well, since dermatology inpatient beds are no longer available in many hospitals. As a consequence, more dermatology patients are managed in the community with a greater role for the community nurse and general practitioner or family doctor. Dermatology liaison nurses play a very important part in making sure that the patients are using their treatment effectively at home and in maintaining the link between the hospital department, the home situation, and the general practitioner. Self-help groups are a valuable resource of support for patients, and there is now much more information available to the public on the recognition and management of skin disease.

Progress has been made in increasing the awareness of the general public and the politicians (who control the resources for health care) of the importance of skin diseases. In countries with minimal medical services there are immense challenges—particularly the need for training medical workers in the community who can recognise and treat the most important conditions. This has a major impact on the suffering and disability from skin diseases. The International Foundation for Dermatology and the pioneering Regional Dermatology Training Centre in Moshi, Tanzania, have set an important lead in this regard.

All the chapters have been revised for this new edition and a number of new illustrations included. A new chapter on tropical dermatology, which was previously included in the "hot climates" Australasian edition, is incorporated. In addition, there is a chapter on dermatology in general practice. Colleagues with special areas of expertise have been generous in giving advice and suggestions for this edition, which I trust will be a means of introducing the reader to a fascinating clinical discipline, covering all age groups and relevant to all areas of medicine.

Edinburgh, 2003, Paul Buxton

1 Introduction

The object of this book is to provide the non-dermatologist with a practical guide to the diagnosis and treatment of skin conditions. One advantage of dealing with skin conditions is that the lesions are easily examined and can be interpreted without the need for complex investigations, although a biopsy may be required to make or confirm the diagnosis. An understanding of the microscopic changes underlying the clinical presentation makes this interpretation easier and more interesting.

In the early chapters the relationship between the clinical presentation and the underlying pathological changes is discussed for a few important conditions, such as psoriasis. These are then used as a model for comparison with other skin diseases. This approach is suitable for skin conditions that present with characteristic lesions.

In other disorders a variety of causes may produce the same type of lesion. In this case it is more helpful to describe the characteristic clinical pattern that results. For example, similar inflamatory changes may result from drug allergy, autoimmune disease, or infection.

Tumours, acne, and leg ulcers are covered as separate subjects, as are diseases of the hair and nails.

The same condition is sometimes dealt with in more than one section, for example, fungal infections are discussed under "Rashes with epidermal changes" and again under "Fungal and yeast infections", giving different perspectives of the same disorder.

Skin lesions are sometimes an indication of internal disease and may be the first clinical sign. For example, the girl in the photograph presented with a rash on her face, made worse by sunlight. She then mentioned that she was aware of lassitude, weight loss, and vague musculoskeletal symptoms which, in conjunction with the appearance of the rash, suggested lupus erythematosus. This was confirmed by further investigations and appropriate treatment was initiated. Other dermatological associations with systemic disease are discussed in the relevant sections.

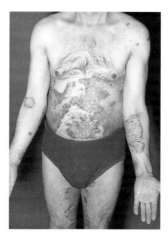

Psoriasis—large legions

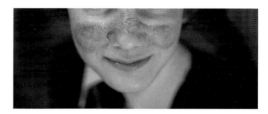

Lupus erythematosus

The significance of skin disease

A large proportion of the population suffers from skin diseases, which make up about 10% of all consultations in primary care in the United Kingdom. However, community studies show that over 20% of the population have a medically significant skin condition and less than 25% of these consulted a doctor.

The skin is not only the largest organ of the body, it also forms a living biological barrier and is the aspect of ourselves we present to the world. It is therefore not surprising that there is great interest in "skin care", with the associated vast cosmetic industry. The impairment of the normal functions of the skin can lead to acute and chronic illness with considerable disability and sometimes a need for hospital treatment.

A wide variety of tumours, both benign and malignant, arise in the skin. Fortunately the majority are harmless and most moles never develop dysplastic change.

Most cancers arising in the skin remain localised and are only invasive locally, but others may metastasise. It is important therefore to recognise the features of benign and malignant tumours, particularly those, such as malignant melanoma, that

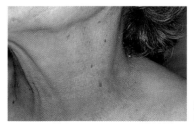

Skin tags—examples of benign tumours

1

can develop widespread metastases. Recognition of typical benign tumours saves the patient unneccessary investigations and the anxiety involved in waiting for results.

Although a wide range of internal diseases produce physical signs in the skin, most skin diseases do not themselves have serious physical effects. However there can be significant psychological effects and problems with personal relationships, employment, and sporting activity. It is therefore important to use what Dr Papworth called "wide angle lenses" in assessing the patient and their disease. So, in addition to concentrating on the skin changes, the overall health and demeanour of the patient should be taken into account. This also means making sure that there are no other signs, such as involvement of the nails, mucous membranes, or other parts of the skin. The general physical condition and psychological state of the patient should be assessed, with more specific examination if indicated.

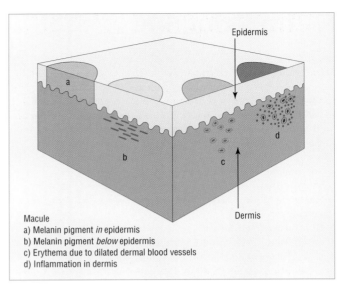

Macule
a) Melanin pigment *in* epidermis
b) Melanin pigment *below* epidermis
c) Erythema due to dilated dermal blood vessels
d) Inflammation in dermis

Section through skin

Descriptive terms

All specialties have their own common terms, and familiarity with a few of those used in dermatology is a great help. The most important are defined below.

Macule
Derived from the Latin for a stain, the term macule is used to describe changes in colour or consistency without any elevation above the surface of the surrounding skin. There may be an increase of melanin, giving a black or blue colour depending on the depth of the pigment. Loss of melanin leads to a white macule. Vascular dilatation and inflammation produce erythema.

Papules and nodules
A papule is a circumscribed, raised lesion, conventionally less than 1 cm in diameter. It may be due to either epidermal or dermal changes.

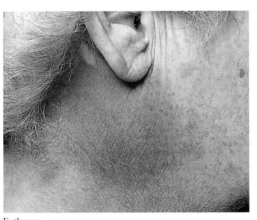

Eythema

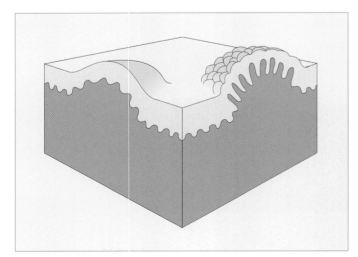

Section through skin with a papule

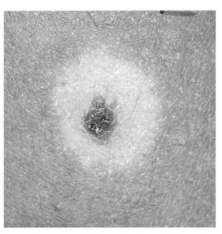

A papule surrounded by a depigmented macule

A nodule is similar to a papule but over 1 cm in diameter.
A vascular papule or nodule is known as an haemangioma.

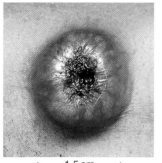
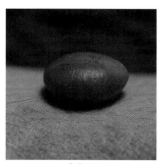

←— 1.5 cm —→

Nodule

←— 0.5 cm —→

Papule (haemangioma)

Plaque

Plaque is one of those terms which conveys a clear meaning to
dermatologists but is often not understood by others. To take it
literally, one can think of a commemorative plaque stuck on
the wall of a building, with a large area relative to its height and
a well defined edge. Plaques are most commonly seen in
psoriasis.

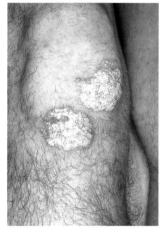

Plaques in psoriasis

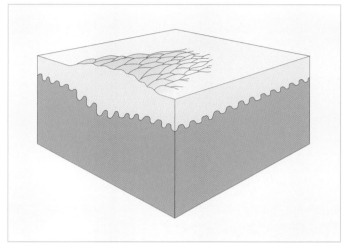

Section through skin with plaque

Vesicles and bullae

Vesicles and bullae are raised lesions that contain fluid. A bulla
is a vesicle larger than 0.5 cm. They may be superficial within
the epidermis or situated in the dermis below it.

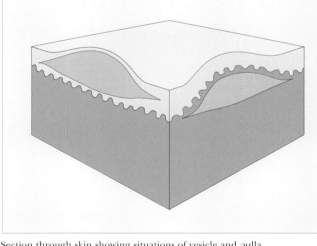

Section through skin showing situations of vesicle and bulla

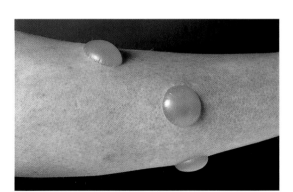

Acute reaction to insect bite—bullae

Lichenification

Lichenification is another term frequently used in
dermatology as a relic of the days of purely descriptive
medicine. Some resemblance to lichen seen on rocks and
trees does occur, with hard thickening of the skin and
accentuated skin markings. It is most often seen as a
result of prolonged rubbing of the skin in localised
areas of eczema.

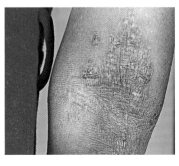

Lichen simplex

Nummular lesions

Nummular literally means a "coin-like" lesion. There is no hard and fast distinction from *discoid* lesions, which are flat disc-like lesions of variable size. It is most often used to describe a type of eczematous lesion.

Pustules

The term pustule is applied to lesions containing purulent material—which may be due to infection, as in the case shown—or sterile pustules, which are seen in pustular psoriasis.

Atrophy

Atrophy refers to loss of tissue which may affect the epidermis, dermis, or subcutaneous fat. Thinning of the epidermis is characterised by loss of the normal skin markings, and there may be fine wrinkles, loss of pigment, and a translucent appearance. There may be other changes as well, such as sclerosis of the underlying connective tissue, telangiectasia, or evidence of diminished blood supply.

Ulceration

Ulceration results from the loss of the whole thickness of the epidermis and upper dermis. Healing results in a scar.

Erosion

An erosion is a superficial loss of epidermis that generally heals without scarring.

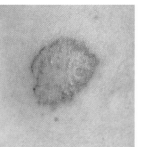
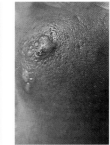

Numular lesion as a response to a vaccination site in the arm

Pustule due to infection

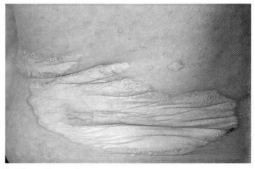

Epidermal atrophy

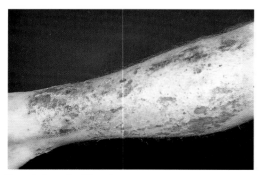

Tropical ulcer

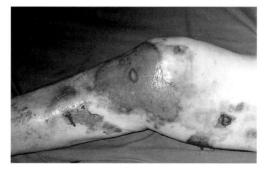

Bullous pemphigoid causing erosion

Excoriation

Excoriation is the partial or complete loss of epidermis as a result of scratching.

Fissuring

Fissures are slits through the whole thickness of the skin.

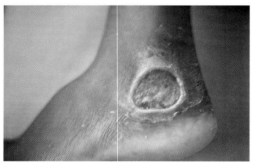

Excoriation of epidermis

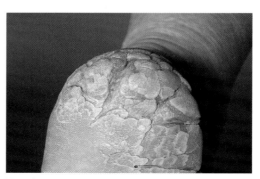

Hyperkeratosis with fissures

Desquamation
Desquamation is the peeling of superficial scales, often following acute inflammation.

Annular lesions
Annular lesions are ring shaped lesions.

Reticulate
The term reticulate means "net-like". It is most commonly seen when the pattern of subcutaneous blood vessels becomes visible.

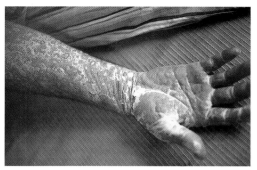

Desquamation

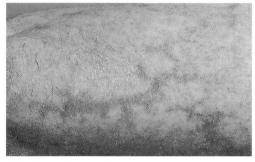

Reticulate pattern on skin

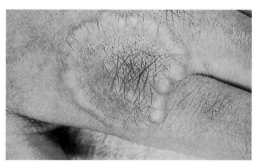

Ring-shaped annular lesion

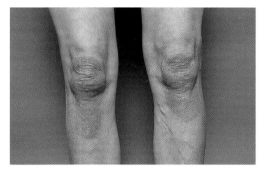

Psoriasis of both legs

Rashes

Approach to diagnosis
A skin rash generally poses more problems in diagnosis than a single, well defined skin lesion such as a wart or tumour. As in all branches of medicine a reasonable diagnosis is more likely to be reached by thinking firstly in terms of broad diagnostic categories rather than specific conditions.

There may have been previous episodes because it is a constitutional condition, such as atopic eczema. In the case of contact dermatitis, regular exposure to a causative agent leads to recurrences that fit with the times of exposure and this is usually apparent from the history. Endogenous conditions such as psoriasis can appear in adults who have had no previous episodes. If there is no family history and several members of the household are affected, a contagious condition, such as scabies, should be considered. A common condition with a familial tendency, such as atopic eczema, may affect several family members at different times.

A simplistic approach to rashes is to clarify them as being from "inside" or "outside". Examples of "inside" or endogenous rashes are atopic eczema or drug rashes, whereas fungal infection or contact dermatitis are "outside" rashes.

Symmetry
Most endogenous rashes affect both sides of the body, as in the atopic child or a man with psoriasis on his knees. Of course, not all exogenous rashes are asymmetrical. A seamstress who uses scissors in her right hand may develop an allergy to metal in this one hand, but a hairdresser or nurse can develop contact dermatitis on both hands.

Diagnosis of rash
- Previous episodes of the rash, particularly in childhood, suggest a constitutional condition such as atopic eczema
- Recurrences of the rash, particularly in specific situations, suggests a contact dermatitis. Similarly a rash that only occurs in the summer months may well have a photosensitive basis
- If other members of the family are affected, particularly without any previous history, there may well be a transmissible condition such as scabies

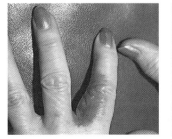

Contact dermatitis as a response to mascara

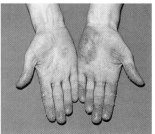

Irritant dermatitis

Distribution

It is useful to be aware of the usual sites of common skin conditions. These are shown in the appropriate chapters. Eruptions that appear only on areas exposed to sun may be entirely or partially due to sunlight. Some are due to a sensitivity to sunlight alone, such as polymorphous light eruption, or a photosensitive allergy to topically applied substances or drugs taken internally.

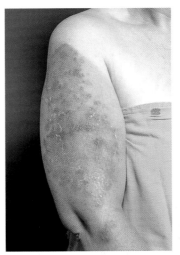

Allergic reaction producing photosensitivity

Morphology

The appearance of the skin lesion may give clues to the underlying pathological process.

The surface may consist of normal epidermis overlying a lesion in the deeper tissues. This is characteristic of many types of erythema in which there is dilatation of the dermal blood vessels associated with inflammation. The skin overlying cysts or tumours in the dermis and deeper tissues is usually normal. Conditions affecting the epidermis will produce several visible changes such as thickening of the keratin layer and scales in psoriasis or a more uniform thickening of the epidermis in areas lichenified by rubbing. An eczematous process is characterised by small vesicles in the epidermis with crusting or fine scaling.

The margin of some lesions is very well defined, as in psoriasis or lichen planus, but in eczema it merges into normal skin.

Blisters or vesicles occur as a result of (a) oedema between the epidermal cells or (b) destruction of epidermal cells or (c) the result of separation of the epidermis from the deeper tissues. Of course, more than one mechanism may occur in the same lesion. Oedema within the epidermis is seen in endogenous eczema, although it may not be apparent clinically, particularly if it is overshadowed by inflammation and crusts. It is also a feature of contact dermatitis.

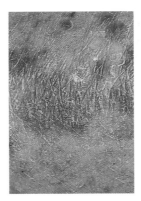

Lesion in deeper tissue with normal epidermis

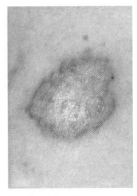

Small vesicles of eczema

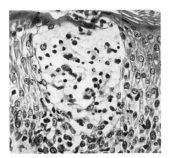

Eczema—intraepidermal vesicle

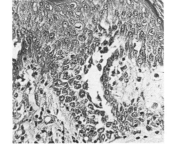

Pemphigus—destruction of epidermal cells

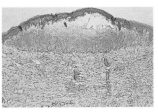

Pemphigoid—blister forming below epidermis

Blisters occur in:

- *viral diseases* such as chickenpox, hand, foot and mouth disease, and herpes simplex
- *bacterial infections* such as impetigo
- eczema and contact dermatitis
- *primary blistering* disorders such as dermatitis herpetiformis, pemphigus and pemphigoid as well as metabolic disorders such as porphyria.

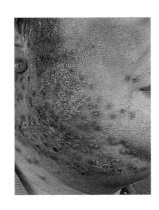

Herpes simplex

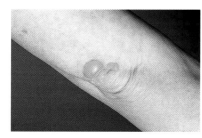

Impetigo

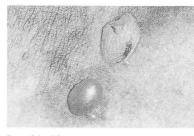

Pemphigoid

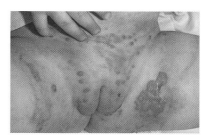

Impetigo

Bullae, blisters over 0.5 cm in diameter, may occur in congenital conditions (such as epidermolysis bullosa), lichen planus, and pemphigoid without much inflammation. However, those forming as a result of vasculitis, sunburn, or an allergic reaction may be associated with pronounced inflammation. In pustular psoriasis there are deeper pustules, which contain polymorphs but are sterile and show little inflammation. Drug rashes can appear as a bullous eruption.

Induration is thickening of the skin due to infiltration of cells, granuloma formation, or deposits of mucin, fat, or amyloid.

Inflammation is indicated by erythema, which may be accompanied by increased temperature if acute—for example, in cellulitis or erythema nodosum. There may be a chronic inflammatory infiltrate in, for example, conditions such as lichen planus or lupus erythematosus.

Assessment of the patient

As well as assessing the clinical changes, the effect of a skin condition on the patient's life and their attitude to it must always be taken into account. For example, severe pustular psoriasis of the hands can be devastating for a self employed electrician and total hair loss from the scalp very distressing for a 16 year old girl.

Fear that a skin condition may be due to cancer or infection is often present and reassurance should always be given whether asked for or not. If there is the possibility of a serious underlying cause that requires further investigation, it is part of good management to answer any questions the patient has and provide an explanation that he or she can understand. It is easy to forget this aspect of medical practice at times.

The significance of occupational factors must be taken into account. In some cases, such as an allergy to hair dyes in a hairdresser, it may be impossible for the patient to continue their job. In other situations the allergy can be easily avoided.

Patients understandably ask whether psoriasis can be cured and often want to know the cause. The cause is unknown and the best answer is that the tendency to develop psoriasis is part of a person's constitution and some factor triggers the development of the clinical lesions. Known factors include physical or emotional stress, local trauma to the skin (Koebner's phenomenon), infection (in guttate psoriasis), drugs (β blockers, lithium, and antimalarial drugs).

To illustrate the use of these basic concepts in the diagnosis of lesions in practice two common skin diseases are considered— *psoriasis*, which affects 1–2% of the population, and *eczema*, an even more common complaint. Both are rashes with distinctive epidermal changes. The difficulty arises with the unusual lesion: Is it a rarity or a variation of a common disease? What should make us consider further investigation? Is it safe to wait and see if it resolves or persists? The usual clinical presentations of psoriasis and eczema are also used as a basis for comparison with variations of the usual pattern and other skin conditions.

A relevant history should be taken in relation to occupational and environmental factors

- Where? Site of initial lesion(s) and subsequent distribution
- How long? Has condition been continuous or intermittent?
- Prognosis—Is it getting better or worse?
- Previous episodes—How long ago? Were they similar? Have there been other skin conditions?
- Who else? Are other members of the family affected? Or colleagues at work or school?
- Other features—Is there itching, burning, scaling, or blisters? Any association with drugs or other illnesses?
- Treatment—By prescription or over the counter? Have prescribed treatments actually been used?

The following points are helpful when examining skin lesions

Distribution
- This may give the essential clue, so a full examination is necessary. For example, there are many possible causes for dry thickened skin on the palms, and finding typical psoriasis on the elbows, knees, and soles may give the diagnosis

Morphology
- Are the lesions dermal or epidermal? Macular (flat) or forming papules? Indurated or forming plaques? With a well defined edge? Forming crusts, scabs, or vesicles?

Pattern
- This is the overall clinical picture of both morphology and distribution. For example, an indeterminate rash may be revealed as pityriasis rosea when the "herald patch" is found

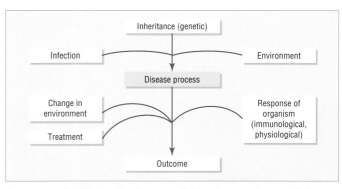

Factors possibly affecting development of skin disease such as psoriasis

---

Further reading

Braun-Falco O, Plewig G, Wolff HH, Winkelmann RK. *Dermatology.* Berlin: Springer-Verlag, 1991

Champion RH, Burton JL, Ebling FJ. *Textbook of dermatology.* 6th ed. Oxford: Blackwell Scientific, 1998

Fitzpatrick TB, Freedberg IM, Eisen AZ, Austen KF, Wolff K. *Dermatology in general medicine.* 4th ed. New York: McGraw-Hill, 1993

Sams WM, Lynch PJ, eds. *Principles and practice of dermatology,* 2nd ed. New York: Churchill Livingstone, 1996

2 Psoriasis

The familiar pink or red lesions with a scaling surface and well defined edge are easily recognised. These changes can be related to the histological appearance:

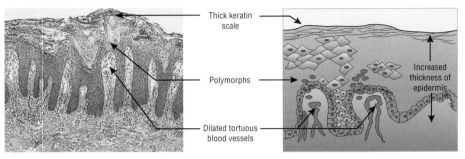

Increased epidermal proliferation—nuclei found … throughout the epidermis

- The increased thickness of the epidermis, presence of nuclei above the basal layer, and thick keratin are related to increased epidermal turnover.
- Because the epidermis is dividing it does not differentiate adequately into normal keratin scales. These are readily removed to reveal the tortuous blood vessels beneath, appearing clinically as "Auspitz sign". The psoriatic plaque can be likened to a brick wall badly built by a workman in too much of a hurry—it may be high but it is easily knocked down.
- The polymorphs that migrate into the epidermis form sterile pustules in pustular psoriasis. These are most commonly seen on the palms and soles.
- The dilated blood vessels can be a main feature, giving the clinical picture of intense erythema.

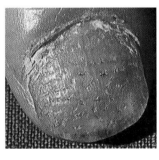

Pitting of the nail

The equivalent changes in the nail cause thickening and "pits" 0.5–1.0 mm in diameter on the surface; these are thought to be due to small areas of psoriatic changes in the upper layer of the nail plate that then fall out. Onycholysis, in which the nail plate is raised up, also occurs in psoriasis.

Clinical appearance

The main characteristics of psoriatic lesions, which reflect the pathological processes listed above, follow.

Plaques consisting of well defined raised areas of psoriasis. These may be few or numerous, covering large areas of the trunk and limbs. Sometimes there are large confluent lesions.

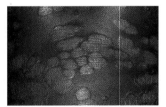

Small lesions

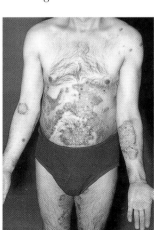

Large lesions

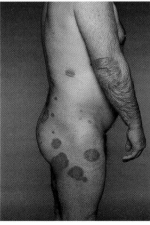

Plaques

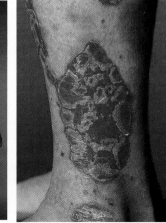

Plaques

Scaling may predominate, giving a thick plaque, which is sometimes likened to limpets on the sea shore, hence the name "rupioid". Scratching the surface produces a waxy appearance—the "tache de bougie" (literally "a line of candle wax").

Erythema may be conspicuous, especially in lesions on the trunk and flexures.

Pustules are rare on the trunk and limbs, but deep seated pustules on the palms and soles are fairly common. In the form of *palmo-plantar pustulosis* they may occur without psoriasiatic lesions elsewhere.

The *size* of the lesions varies from a few millimetres to very extensive plaques.

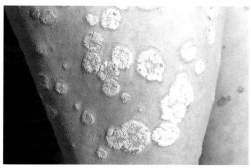
Rupoid lesions

The typical patient

Psoriasis usually occurs in early adult life, but the onset can be at any time from infancy to old age, when the appearance is often atypical.

The following factors in the history may help in making a diagnosis:

- There may be a family history—if one parent has psoriasis 16% of the children will have it, if both parents, the figure is 50%.
- The onset can occur after any type of stress, including infection, trauma, or childbirth.
- The lesions may first appear at sites of minor trauma—Koebner's phenomenon.
- The lesions usually clear on exposure to the sun.
- Typically, psoriasis does not itch.
- There may be associated arthropathy—affecting either the fingers and toes or a single large joint.

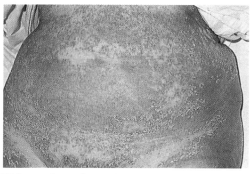
Widespread pustular psoriasis

Clinical presentation

Patients usually present with lesions on the elbows, knees, and scalp. The trunk may have plaques of variable size and which are sometimes annular. Patients with psoriasis show Koebner's phenomenon with lesions developing in areas of skin trauma such as scars or minor scratches. Normal everyday trauma such as handling heavy machinery may produce hyperkeratotic lesions on the palms. In the scalp there is scaling, sometimes producing very thick accretions. Erythema often extends beyond the hair margin. The nails show "pits" and also thickening with separation of the nail from the nail bed (oncholysis).

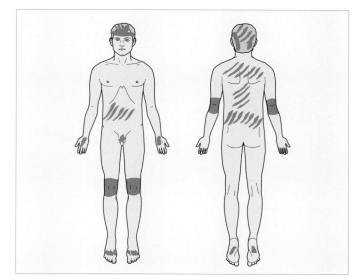
Common patterns of distribution in psoriasis

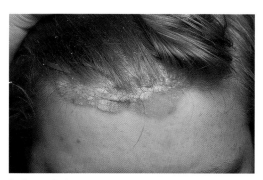
Scalp psoriasis

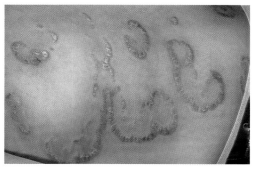
Annular lesions

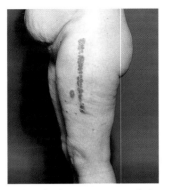

Koebner's phenomenon: psoriasis
in surgical scar

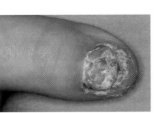

Psoriasis of the nail

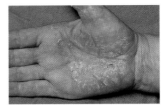

Psoriasis of the hand

Guttate psoriasis—from the Latin *gutta*, a drop—consists of widespread small pink macules that look like drops of paint. It usually occurs in adolescents and often follows an acute β haemolytic streptococcal infection. There may be much distress to both parent and child when a previously healthy adolescent erupts in spots. Fortunately it also resolves quite rapidly.

Pustular lesions occur as either chronic deep seated lesions or generalised pustular psoriasis.

Chronic deep seated lesions occur on the palms and soles with surrounding erythema which develops a brown colour and scaling. It is important to reassure the patient that, despite their appearance, these pustules are not infectious—they consist of sterile collections of polymorphs.

These lesions occur in an older age group than psoriasis, and psoriasis may not be present elsewhere. It is more common in smokers. *Acrodermatitis pustulosa* is a variant that occurs in a younger age group in which there are pustules and inflammation arround the nails and the fingertips.

Generalised pustular psoriasis is uncommon. Pustules develop in association with erythema. It may be precipitated by the use of steroids.

Flexural psoriasis produces well defined erythematous areas in the axillae and groins and beneath the breasts. Scaling is minimal or absent. It must be distinguished from a fungal infection and it is wise to send specimens for mycology if there is any doubt.

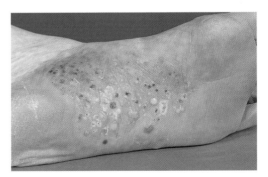

Guttate psoriasis

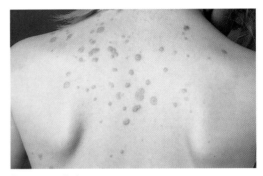

Pustules on the foot

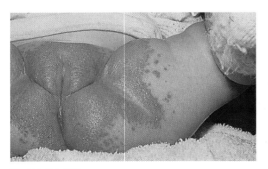

Napkin psoriasis

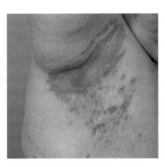

Flexural psoriasis

Napkin psoriasis in children may present with typical psoriatic lesions or a more diffuse erythematous eruption with exudative rather than scaling lesions.

Erythrodermic psoriasis is a serious, even life threatening, condition with erythema affecting nearly the whole of the skin. Diagnosis may not be easy as the characteristic scaling of psoriasis is absent, although this usually precedes the erythroderma. Less commonly the erythema develops suddenly without preceding lesions. There is a considerable increase in cutaneous blood flow, heat loss, metabolism, and water loss.

It is important to distinguish between the *stable*, chronic, plaque type of psoriasis, which is unlikely to develop exacerbations and responds to tar, dithranol, and ultraviolet treatment, and the more *acute* erythematous type, which is unstable and likely to spread rapidly. The use of tar, dithranol, or ultraviolet light can irritate the skin and will make it more widespread and inflamed.

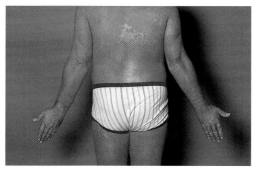
Erytherodermic psoriasis

Joint disease in psoriasis

Patients with seronegative arthropathy of the non-rheumatoid type show double the normal (2%) incidence of psoriasis. Psoriatic arthropathy commonly affects the distal interphalangeal joints, sparing the metacarpophalangeal joints, and is usually asymmetrical. Radiological changes include a destructive arthropathy with deformity. Rheumatoid nodules are absent. The sex ratio is equal but a few patients develop a "rheumatoid-like" arthropathy, which is more common in women than in men. A third rare group have arthritic changes in the larger joints, where there is considerable resorption of bone. Other members of the families of those with psoriatic arthropathy are affected in 40% of cases.

There may be pustular psoriasis of the fingers and toes associated with arthropathy which can be sufficiently severe to immobilise the patient.

Both psoriatic arthropathy and Reiter's syndrome are associated with the presence of HLA B27. Reiter's syndrome is characterised by polyarthritis and the development of urethritis, inflammatory changes in the conjunctivae, and skin lesions including pustulosis hyperkeratosis of the soles.

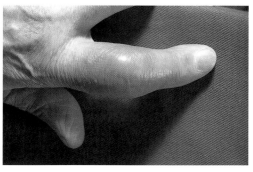
Acute arthropathy

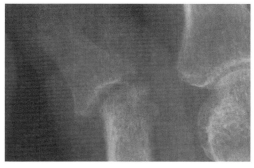
Acute arthropathy—*X* ray signs

Causes of psoriasis

The cause is unknown but there is an inherited predisposition. The strong genetic influence may result from a single dominant gene with poor penetrance or a number of genetic influences. Other factors such as local trauma, general illness and stress are also involved, so the cause of psoriasis is best regarded as being multifactorial. HLA-Cw6 is the phenotype most strongly associated with psoriasis, particularly the early onset variety in which hereditary factors seem to play the greatest part. There is an increase in HLA expression in psoriatic arthropathy.

Local trauma, acute illness, and stress may be factors in causing the appearance of clinical lesions. β Haemolytic streptococcal throat infection is a common precipitating factor in guttate psoriasis. Antimalarial drugs, lithium, and β blockers can make psoriasis worse. There is evidence that psoriasis occurs more readily and is more intractable in patients with a high intake of alcohol. Smoking is associated with palmo-plantar pustulosis.

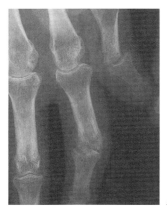
Acute arthropathy—*X* ray signs

There is evidence that both hormonal and immunological mechanisms are involved at a cellular level. The raised concentrations of metabolites of arachodonic acid in the affected skin of people with psoriasis are related to the clinical changes. Prostaglandins cause erythema, whereas leukotrienes (LTB4 and 12 HETE) cause neutrophils to accumulate. The common precursor of these factors is phospholipase A2, which is influenced by calmodulin, a cellular receptor protein for calcium. Both phospholipase A2 and calmodulin concentrations are raised in psoriatic lesions.

T helper lymphocytes have been found in the dermis as well as antibodies to the basal cell nuclei of psoriatic skin. In addition, dermal factors contribute to the development of psoriatic lesions.

The detailed treatment of psoriasis is covered in the next chapter. The only point to be made here is the importance of encouraging a positive attitude with expectation of improvement but not a permanent cure, since psoriasis can recur at any time. Some patients are unconcerned about very extensive lesions whereas to others the most minor lesions are a catastrophe.

Further reading

Farber EM. *Psoriasis.* Amsterdam: Elsevier, 1987

Fry L. *An atlas of psoriasis.* London: Parthenon Publications, 1992

Mier PD, Van de Kerkhof PC. *Textbook of psoriasis.* Edinburgh: Churchill Livingstone, 1986

Roenigk HH, Maibach HI. *Psoriasis.* Basle: Dekker, 1991

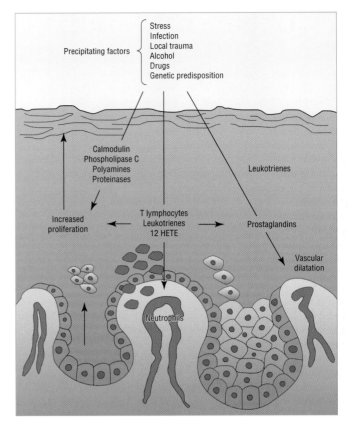

Hormonal and immunological mechanisms and dermal factors involved in the development of psoriasis

3 Treatment of psoriasis

It vanished quite slowly, beginning with the end of the tail, and ending with the grin, which remained some time after the rest of it had gone.
Lewis Carroll, *Alice in Wonderland*

To ignore the impact of the condition on the patient's life is to fail in treating psoriasis. Like the Cheshire cat that Alice met, it tends to clear slowly and the last remaining patches are often the hardest to clear. This is frustrating enough, but there is also the knowledge that it will probably recur and need further tedious courses of treatment, so encouragement and support are an essential part of treatment.

In an attempt to quantify the impact of psoriasis on the life of the individual patient the Psoriasis Disability Index (PDI) has been developed. This takes the form of a questionnaire and covers all aspects of the patient's work, personal relationships, domestic situation, and recreational activities. It can be helpful in assessing the effectiveness of treatment as perceived by the patient.

Patients understandably ask whether psoriasis can be cured and often want to know the cause. The cause is unknown and the best answer is that the tendency to develop psoriasis is part of an affected person's constitution and some factor triggers the development of the clinical lesions. Known factors include physical or emotional stress, local trauma to the skin (Koebner's phenomenon), infection (in guttate psoriasis), drugs (β blockers, lithium, and antimalarial drugs).

Treatment comprises ointments and pastes, systemic drugs, or various forms of ultraviolet light. The treatment should suit the type of psoriasis. The age and health of the patient, social and occupational factors need to be taken into consideration. The motivation of the individual patient is also important.

The preparations mentioned in the text are listed in the formulary in chapter 26. It is estimated that 80% of patients with psoriasis do not consult a doctor, as the lesions are minimal.

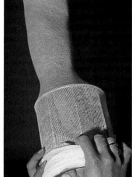
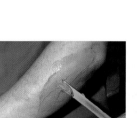

Preparation applied to affected area (left). Application of stockinette (right)

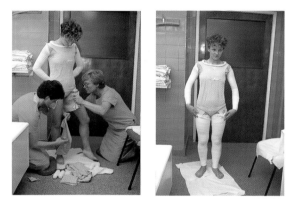

Bandages being applied to larger areas (left). Patient now prepared for contact treatment (right)

Treatment of psoriasis

Type of psoriasis	Treatment	Alternative treatment
Stable plaque psoriasis	Tar preparations Calcipotriol + topical steroids Tacalcitol Ultraviolet B (TL 01)	Short contact dithranol
Extensive stable plaques	As above. If not responding: Ultraviolet B (TL01) psoralen with ultraviolet A + etretinate	Methotrexate Ciclosporin A Tacrolimus
Widespread small plaque	Ultraviolet B	Tar
Guttate psoriasis	Emollients then ultraviolet B	Weak tar preparations
Facial psoriasis	1% hydrocortisone ointment	
Flexural psoriasis	Local mild to moderate strength steroids + antifungal	
Pustular psoriasis of hands and feet	Moderate to potent strength topical steroids	Acitretin
Acute erythrodermic, unstable, or general pustular psoriasis	Inpatient treatment Short term local steroids for acutely inflamed lesions	Methotrexate Acitretin Ciclosporin or other immunosuppressants

Local treatment

Local treatments entail the use of ointments and pastes, usually containing tar in various forms. It is much easier to apply them in hospital than at home if patients can make the time for hospital visits. Inpatient treatment can be more intensive and closely regulated; it also has the advantage of taking the patient completely away from the stresses of the everyday environment. In some units a "five day ward" enables patients to return home at weekends, which is particularly important for parents with young children.

Coal tar preparations are safe and effective for the stable plaque-type psoriasis but will irritate acute, inflamed areas. However, tar may not be strong enough for thicker hyperkeratotic lesions. Salicylic acid, which helps dissolve keratin, can be used in conjunction with tar for thick plaques. Refined coal tar extracts can be used for less severe areas of psoriasis.

Ichthammol, prepared from shale rather than coal tar, is less irritating and has a soothing effect on inflamed skin. It is therefore useful for "unstable" or inflamed psoriasis, when tar would not be tolerated.

Dithranol, obtained originally from the Goa tree in south India, is now made synthetically. It can easily irritate or burn the skin, so it has to be used carefully and should be kept from contact with normal skin as far as possible. For hospital treatment pastes are used and the lesions surrounded by petroleum jelly to protect the normal skin. Dithranol creams can be used at home—they are applied for 30 minutes and then washed off. A low concentration (0·1%) is used initially and gradually increased to 1% or 2% as necessary. All dithranol preparations are irritants and produce a purple-brown staining that clears in time. If used in the scalp dithranol stains red or fair hair purple.

Emollients soften dry skin and relieve itching. They are a useful adjunct to tar or dithranol.

Corticosteroid preparations produce an initial clearing of psoriasis, but there is rapid relapse when they are withdrawn and tachyphylaxis (increasing amounts of the drug having a diminishing effect) occurs. Strong topical steroids should be avoided. Only weak preparations should be used on the face but moderately potent steroids can be used elsewhere:
(a) if there are only a few small lesions of psoriasis;
(b) if there is persistent chronic psoriasis of the palms, soles, and scalp (in conjunction with tar paste, which is applied on top of the steroid at night); and (c) in the treatment of psoriasis of the ears, flexures, and genital areas. In flexural psoriasis secondary infection can occur and steroid preparations combined with antibiotics and antifungal drugs should be used, such as Terra-Cortril with nystatin and Trimovate.

Systemic corticosteroids should not be used, except in life threatening erythroderma, because of the inevitable "rebound" that occurs when the dose is reduced. The management of psoriasis in patients taking steroids for an unrelated condition may require inpatient or regular outpatient attendances to clear the skin lesions.

Calcipotriol and *tacalcitol*, vitamin D analogues, are calmodulin inhibitors used topically for mild or moderate plaque psoriasis. They are non-staining creams that are easy to use but can cause irritation. Sometimes a plateau effect is seen with the treatment becoming less effective after an initial response. If so, other agents, such as tar preparations, have to be used as well to clear the lesions completely. It is important not to exceed the maximum recommended dose so as to prevent changes in calcium metabolism.

Short contact dithranol

Indications
- Stable plaque psoriasis on the trunk and limbs

Suitable preparations
- Those available are in a range of concentrations such as Dithocream (0·1%, 0·25%, 0·5%, 1·0%, 2·0%) or Anthranol (0·4%, 1·0%, 2·0%)

Method
- Start with the lowest concentration and increase strength every five to six days if there are no problems
- Apply cream to affected areas and then wash it off completely 20–30 minutes later
- Apply a bland emollient immediately after treatment

Cautions
- Do not apply to inflamed plaques, flexures, or the face
- Avoid contact of the dithranol with clothing and rinse the bath well after use to avoid staining
- Never leave the cream on for longer than 30 minutes (60 minutes is not twice as effective)

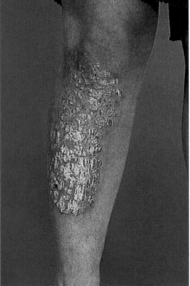

Psoriasis suitable for short contact dithranol treatment

Ultraviolet treatment (phototherapy)

Ultraviolet B is short wavelength ultraviolet light and is used for widespread thin lesions or guttate psoriasis. The dose has to be accurately controlled to give enough radiation to clear the skin without burning. Recently, "narrow waveband" ultraviolet B treatment has been developed, which increases the therapeutic effect and diminishes burning. It can be used instead of psoralen with ultraviolet A in many cases.

Ultraviolet A is long wavelength ultraviolet light, which activates psoralens in the skin. This results in diminished DNA synthesis and hence reduced epidermal turnover. The combination of psoralen with ultraviolet A is known as PUVA therapy: a dose of 8-methoxypsoralen (8MOP), 0·6–0·8 mg/kg body weight, is taken one to two hours before treatment. 5-Methoxypsoralen is also used, particularly in patients develop itching or nausea with 8MOP.

Other long term cumulative side effects of ultraviolet treatment include premature ageing of the skin, lentigenes, and eventually cutaneous malignancies. For this reason the total cumulative dose is kept below 1000 Joules.

After medical assessment treatment is given two or three times a week, with gradually increasing doses of ultraviolet A. Once the psoriasis has cleared maintenance treatments can be continued once every two or three weeks. Protective goggles are worn during treatment with ultraviolet A and dark glasses for 24 hours after each treatment. The glasses are tested for their effectiveness in screening ultraviolet A light.

A variable degree of erythema and itching may occur after treatment. Longer term side effects include a slight risk of epitheliomas developing, premature ageing of the skin, and cataract formation (which can be prevented by wearing ultraviolet A filtering goggles during and after treatment). The total cumulative dosage is carefully monitored and kept as low as possible to reduce the risk of side effects.

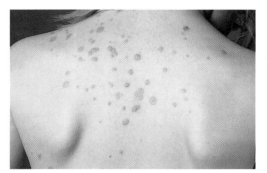

Guttate psoriasis suitable for ultraviolet B treatment

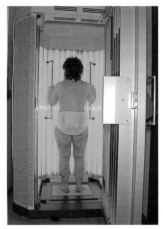

Ultraviolet B cabinet

Systemic treatment

Extensive and inflamed psoriasis that is resistant to local treatment may require systemic treatment. A number of antimetabolite drugs (such as azathioprine and hydroxyurea) and immunosuppressive drugs (such as ciclosporin A) are effective, but the most widely used are methotrexate and acitretin.

Methotrexate inhibits folic acid synthesis during the S phase of mitosis and diminishes epidermal turnover in the lesions of psoriasis. Because it is hepatotoxic liver function has to be assessed initially and at regular intervals during treatment. The dosage must be monitored, and when a total of 1·5 g is reached a liver biopsy is indicated to exclude significant liver damage.

Although it is rare, bone marrow suppression can occur insidiously and rapidly in some patients. In order to detect this an initial test dose is followed by a full blood count. If this gives normal results a weekly dose of 7·5–15 mg is used. As it is excreted in the urine, the dose must be reduced if renal function is impaired. Aspirin and sulphonamides diminish plasma binding.

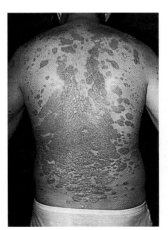

Before phototherapy

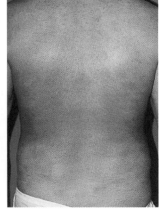

After phototherapy

Methotrexate may interact with barbiturates, para-aminobenzoic acid, phenytoin, probenecid, phenylbutazone, oral contraceptives, and colchicine.

Acitretin is a vitamin A derivative that can be prescribed only in hospital in the United Kingdom. It is useful in pustular psoriasis and has some effect on other types of psoriasis. However, the effect is increased when combined with PUVA. Minor side effects include drying of the mucous membranes, crusting in the nose, itching, thinning of the hair, and erythema of the palms and nail folds. These are usually not severe and settle when treatment stops. More serious side effects include hepatotoxicity and raised lipid concentrations. Liver function tests and serum lipid (cholesterol and triglyceride) concentrations have to be carefully monitored. Etretinate is teratogenic and should only be taken by women during reproductive years if effective contraception is used during treatment and for two years afterwards, as the half life is 70–100 days.

Ciclosporin A is an immunosuppressant widely used following organ transplantation. It is effective in suppressing the inflammatory types of psoriasis. Blood tests should be carried out before starting treatment, particularly serum creatinine, urea, and electrolytes, as ciclosporin A can interfere with renal function.

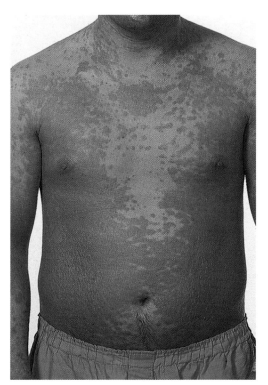

Erythematous psoriasis suitable for methotrexate treatment, having failed to respond to phototherapy

Further reading

Lowe NJ. *Managing your psoriasis.* London: Master Media, 1993
Lowe NJ. *Practical psoriasis therapy*, 2nd ed. St Louis: Mosby, 1992

Psoriasis of the scalp

This condition can be very difficult to clear, particularly if there are thick scales

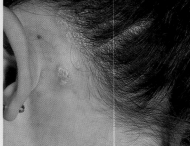

Scalp psoriasis

- 3% salicylic acid in a suitable base and left on for four to six hours or overnight and then washed out with a tar shampoo
- Dithranol preparations are effective but will tint blonde or red hair purple
- Steroid preparations can be used to control itching

4   Eczema and dermatitis

The terms eczema and dermatitis are interchangeable, covering a wide variety of conditions from the child with atopic eczema to the adult with an allergy to cement. If patients are told they have dermatitis they may assume that it is related to their employment with the implication that they may be eligible for compensation. It is not unusual for industrial workers to ask "Is it dermatitis, doctor?", meaning "is it due to my job?"

Clinical appearance

Eczema is an inflammatory condition of the skin characterised by groups of vesicular lesions with a variable degree of exudate and scaling. In some cases dryness and scaling predominate, with little inflammation. In more acute cases there may be considerable inflammation and vesicle formation, in keeping with the Greek for "to boil out", from which the word eczema is derived. Sometimes the main feature may be blisters that become very large.

Eczema commonly itches and the clinical appearance may be modified by scratching, which with time may produce lichenification (thickening of the skin with increased skin markings). Also as a result of scratching the skin surface may be broken and have excoriations, exudate, and secondary infection.

Pathology

The characteristic change is oedema between the cells of the epidermis, known as *spongiosus*, leading to formation of vesicles. The whole epidermis becomes thickened with an increased keratin layer. A variable degree of vasodilatation in the dermis and an inflammatory infiltrate may be present.

Types of eczema

The many causes of eczema are not consistently related to the distribution and clinical appearance. In general there are either external factors acting on the skin producing inflammatory changes or it is an endogenous condition. It is important to remember there can be more than one cause—for example, in atopic eczema or varicose eczema on the ankle an allergic reaction may develop to the treatments used.

Atopic eczema affects mainly the flexor surfaces of the elbows and knees as well as the face and neck. To a variable degree it can affect the trunk as well.

The typical patient with atopic eczema is a fretful, scratching child with eczema that varies in severity, often from one hour to the next. In the older child or adult, eczema is more chronic and widespread and its occurrence is often related to stress. Atopic eczema is common, affecting 3% of all infants, and runs a chronic course with variable remissions. It normally clears during childhood but may continue into adolescence and adult life as a chronic disease. It is often associated with asthma and rhinitis. Sufferers from atopic eczema often have a family history of the condition.

Variants of atopic eczema are pityriasis alba—white patches on the face of children with a fair complexion—and chronic juvenile plantar dermatosis—dry cracked skin of the forefoot in children. This does not affect the interdigital spaces and is not due to a fungal infection.

Eczema herpeticum. Children with atopic eczema are particularly prone to herpes virus infection, which may be life

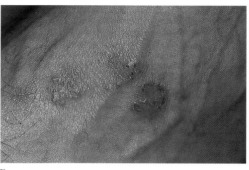

Eczema

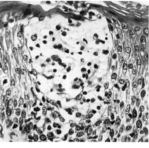

Pathology of eczema

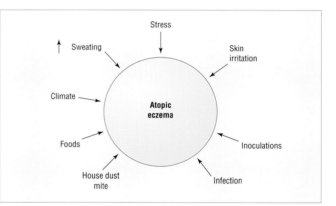

Factors leading to development of atopic eczema

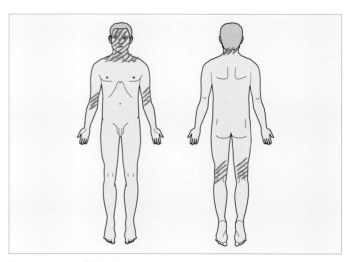

Atopic eczema—distribution

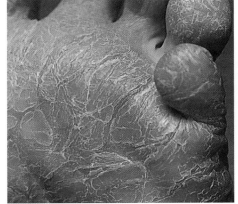

Atopic eczema

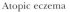

Plantar dermatosis

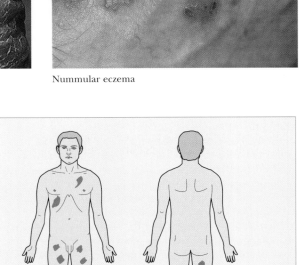

Nummular eczema

threatening. Close contact with adults with "cold sores" should therefore be avoided.

Nummular eczema appears as coin shaped lesions on legs and trunk.

Stasis eczema occurs around the ankles, where there is impaired venous return.

Paget's disease of the breast. Whereas bilateral eczema of the nipples and areolae occur in women, any unilateral, persistent, areas of dermatitis in this region may be caused by Paget's disease, in which there is underlying carcinoma of the ducts. In such cases a biopsy is essential.

Lichen simplex is a localised area of lichenification produced by rubbing.

Neurodermatitis is a term often used synonymously with lichen simplex. It is also used to describe generalised dryness and itching of the skin, usually in those with atopic eczema.

Asteatotic eczema occurs in older people with a dry, "crazypaving" pattern, particularly on the legs.

Pompholyx is itching vesicles on the fingers, with lesions on the palms and soles in some patients.

Infection can modify the presentation of any type of eczema or contact dermatitis.

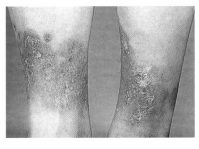

Nummular eczema—distribution

Classification of eczema

Endogenous (constitutional) eczema	Exogenous (contact) eczema	Secondary changes
Atopic	Irritant	Lichen simplex
Nummular or discoid	Allergic	Neurodermatitis
Pompholyx	Photodermatitis	Asteatosis
Stasis		Pompholyx
Seborrhoeic (discussed later)		Infection

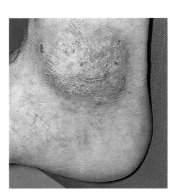

Stasis eczema

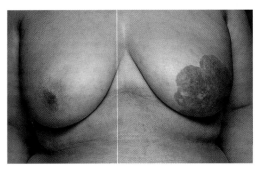

Paget's disease of the nipple

Lichen simplex

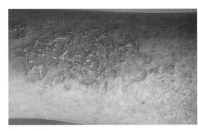

Asteatosis

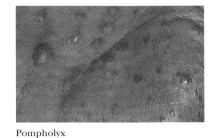

Pompholyx

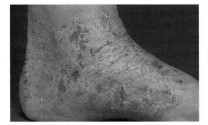

Infected eczema

Contact dermatitis

The skin normally performs its function as a barrier very effectively. If this is overcome by substances penetrating the epidermis an inflammatory response may occur leading to epidermal damage. These changes may be due to either (a) an allergic response to a specific substance acting as a sensitiser or (b) a simple irritant effect. An understanding of the difference between these reactions is helpful in the clinical assessment of contact dermatitis.

Common sources of allergic contact dermatitis

- Jewellery, clothing, wristwatch, scissors, cooking utensils
- Cement, leather
- Hair dyes, tights, shoes
- Rubber gloves and boots
- Creams, ointments, cosmetics
- Nickel—and cobalt occasionally
- Chromate
- Paraphenylenediamine—used in hair dyes
- Rubber preservative chemicals
- Preservatives (parabenz, quarternium), balsam of Peru, fragrances, lanolin, neomycin, benzocaine in medicated ointments

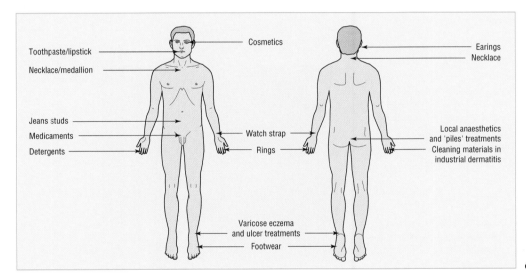

Contact dermatitis—common sources

Allergic contact dermatitis

The characteristics of allergic dermatitis are:

- Previous exposure to the substance concerned.
- 48–96 hours between contact and the development of changes in the skin.
- Activation of previously sensitised sites by contact with the same allergen elsewhere on the body.
- Persistence of the allergy for many years.

The explanation of the sequence of events in a previously sensitised individual is as follows: The antigen penetrates the epidermis and is picked up by a Langerhans cell sensitised to it. It is then transported to the regional lymph node where the paracortical region produces a clone of T cells specifically programmed to react to that antigen. The sensitised T cells accumulate at the site of the antigen and react with it to produce an inflammatory response. This takes 48 hours and is amplified by interleukins that provide a feedback stimulus to the production of further sensitised T cells.

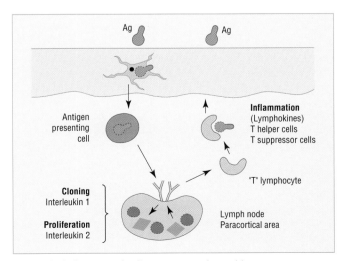

Immunological response leading to contact dermatitis

Allergic contact dermatitis can be illustrated by the example of an individual with an allergy to nickel who has previously reacted to a wrist watch. Working with metal objects that contain nickel leads to dermatitis on the hands and also a flare up at the site of previous contact with the watch. The skin clears on holiday but the dermatitis recurs two days after the person returns to work.

Sensitisers in leg ulcer treatments
- Neomycin
- Lanolin (wool alcohol)
- Formaldehyde
- Tars
- Chinaform (the "C" of many proprietary steroids)

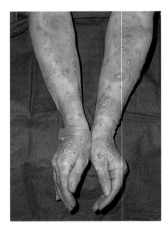
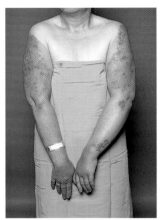

Allergic response to sulfapyridine

Allergic response to Solarcaine and sun

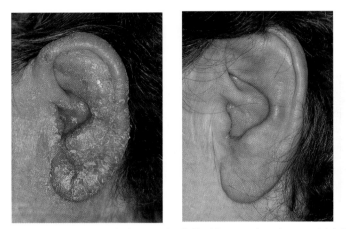

Allergic response to topical neomycin (left). After stopping ointment (right)

Irritant contact dermatitis
This has a much less defined clinical course and is caused by a wide variety of substances with no predictable time interval between contact and the appearance of the rash. Dermatitis occurs soon after exposure and the severity varies with the quantity, concentration, and length of exposure to the substance concerned. Previous contact is not required, unlike allergic dermatitis where previous sensitisation is necessary.

Photodermatitis
Photodermatitis, caused by the interaction of light and chemical absorbed by the skin, occurs in areas exposed to light. It may be due to (a) drugs taken internally, such as sulphonamides, phenothiazines, and dimethylchlortetracycline, or (b) substances in contact with the skin, such as topical antihistamines, local anaesthetics, cosmetics, and antibacterials.

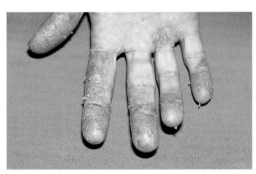

Allergic response to dithranol

Morphology
The clinical appearance of both allergic and irritant contact dermatitis may be similar, but there are specific changes that help in differentiating them. An acute allergic reaction tends to produce erythema, oedema, and vesicles. The more chronic lesions are often lichenified. Irritant dermatitis may present as slight scaling and itching or extensive epidermal damage resembling a superficial burn, as the child in the illustration shows.

Pathology
The reaction to specific allergens leads to a typical eczematous reaction with oedema separating the epidermal cells and blister formation. In irritant dermatitis there may also be eczematous changes but also non-specific inflammation, thickening of keratin, and pyknotic, dead epidermal cells.

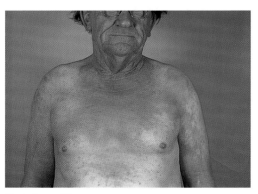

Photodermatitis

The distribution of the skin changes is often helpful. For example, an itchy rash on the waist may be due to an allergy to rubber in the waistband of underclothing or a metal fastener. Gloves or the rubber lining of goggles can cause a persisting dermatitis. An irritant substance often produces a more diffuse eruption, as shown by the patient who developed itching and redness from dithranol.

An allergy to medications used for treating leg ulcers is a common cause of persisting dermatitis on the leg.

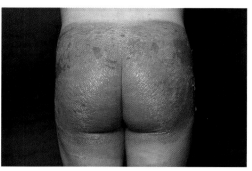

Acute irritant dermatitis

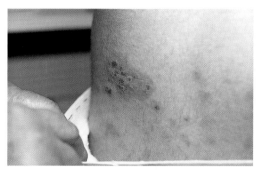

Allergic response to elastic in underpants

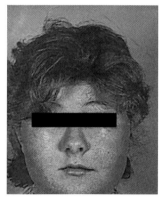

Allergic reaction to cosmetics

Substances commonly causing allergic occupational dermatitis

- Chromate—in cement and leather
- Biocides, for example, formaldehyde and isothiazolinones, used in cutting oils in engineering
- Epoxy resins (uncured monomers)
- Rubber chemicals
- Hair dressing chemicals—particularly dyes and setting lotions
- Plant allergens

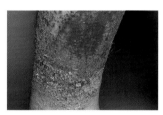

Allergic reaction to epoxy resin

Patch testing

Patch testing is used to determine the substances causing contact dermatitis. The concentration used is critical. If it is too low there may be no reaction, giving a false negative result, and if it is too high it may produce an irritant reaction, which is interpreted as showing an allergy (false positive). Another possible danger is the induction of an allergy by the test substance. The optimum concentration and best vehicle have been found for most common allergens, which are the basis of the "battery" of tests used in most dermatology units.

The test patches are left in place for 48 hours then removed, the sites marked, and any positive reactions noted. A further examination is carried out at 96 hours to detect any further reactions.

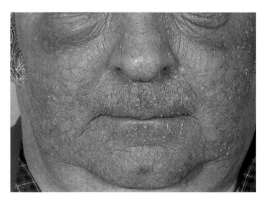

Acutely infected eczema

It is most important not to put a possible causative substance on the skin in a random manner without proper dilution and without control patches. The results will be meaningless and irritant reactions, which are unpleasant for the patient, may occur.

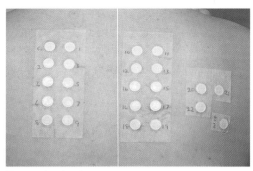

Test patches in place

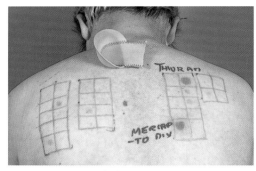

Positive reactions marked

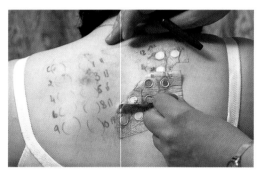

Patches being removed after 48 hours

Occupational dermatitis

Dermatitis, which is simply inflammation of the skin, can arise as a result of:

- Inherited tendency to eczema (atopy)
- Contact dermatitis, which may be either irritant or allergic
- Infection.

In the workplace, all three factors may contribute to dermatitis. For example, a student nurse or trainee hairdresser is exposed to water, detergents, and other factors that will exacerbate any pre-existing eczema. In addition, there may be specific allergies and, as a result of the broken skin, secondary infection can occur making the situation even worse. The following points are helpful in determining the role of occupational causes.

- If the dermatitis first occurred during employment or with a change of employment and had not been present before, then occupational factors are more likely.
- If the condition generally clears during holidays and when away from the workplace, this suggests an occupational cause, but chronic irritant dermatitis may persist when the patient is away from the workplace.
- If there is exposure to substances that are known to induce dermatitis and protective measures are inadequate at the workplace then an occupational cause is likely.
- If secondary infection is present, this can keep a dermatitis active even when away from the workplace and sometimes allergen exposure continues at home; for example, an allergy

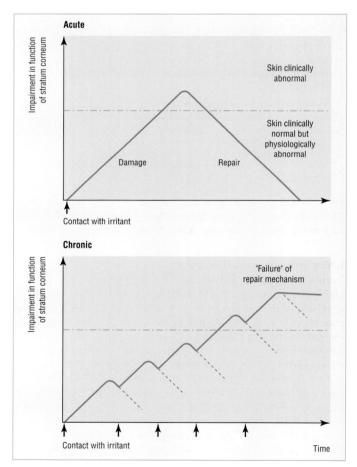

Progression of acute and chronic dermatitis

to rubber gloves at work will also occur when rubber gloves are used for domestic work at home.

Whatever the cause of the dermatitis, the end result may seem the same clinically, because the inflammation and blisters of atopic eczema may be indistinguishable from an allergic reaction to rubber gloves. Generally, contact dermatitis is more common on the dorsal surface of the hands whereas atopic eczema occurs on the palms and sides of the fingers.

Irritant contact dermatitis can occur acutely as mentioned above and there is usually a definite history of exposure to irritating chemicals.

Chronic irritant dermatitis can be harder to assess as it develops insidiously in many cases. Often it starts with episodes of transient inflammation that clear up, but with each successive episode the damage becomes worse with an escalation of inflammatory changes that eventually become chronic and fixed.

Once chronic damage has occurred the skin is vulnerable to any further irritation, so the condition may flare up in the future even after removal of the causative factors. Individuals with atopic eczema are particularly liable to develop chronic irritant dermatitis and secondary infection is an additional factor.

Allergic contact dermatitis occurs as an allergic reaction to specific substances. As this involves a cell mediated response the inflammatory reaction occurs about two days after exposure and once the allergy is present further exposure will inevitably produce a reaction. Some substances are much more likely to produce an allergy, such as epoxy resin monomer, than others, such as cement, which characteristically requires exposure over many years before an allergy develops. In addition to the capacity of the substance to produce an allergic reaction, individuals also vary considerably in the capacity to develop allergies.

Immediate type sensitivity is sometimes seen as a reaction to food protein and sensitivity to latex gloves. This can produce a very severe reaction, particularly in atopic individuals.

The itching skin (pruritus)

It is sometimes very difficult to help a patient with a persistently itching skin, particularly if there is no apparent cause. Pruritus is a general term for itching skin, whatever the reason.

Itching with skin manifestations

Eczema is associated with itching due to the accumulation of fluid between the epidermal cells that are thought to produce stretching of the nerve fibres. As a result of persistent scratching there is often lichenification which conceals the original underlying areas with eczema. Exposure to irritants and persistent allergic reactions can produce intense itching and should always be considered.

"Allergic reactions" due to external agents often cause intense itching. Systemic allergic reactions such as a fixed drug eruption, erythema multiforme, and vasculitis are less likely to cause pruritus.

Psoriasis, which characteristically has hyperkeratotic plaques, usually does not itch but sometimes there can be considerable itching. Occasionally this is due to secondary infection of breaks in the skin surface.

Lichen planus presents with groups of flat-topped papules which often cause an intense itch. Blistering disorders of the skin may itch.

In *herpes simplex* there is usually burning and itching in the early stages.

Treatment of occupational dermatitis
The exact cause of the dermatitis should be identified as far as possible. It is important to ascertain exactly what an individual's job entails; for example, a worker in a plastics factory had severe hand dermatitis but the only positive result on patch testing was to nickel. On visiting the factory it became clear that the cause was a nickel plated handle that he used several thousand times a day and not the plastic components that the machine was making. It is also important to assess the working environment because exposure to damp and irritants (for example, on an oil rig or in a coal mine) can irritate the skin.

If occupational factors are suspected, then a full assessment and investigation in a dermatology department is important as the patient's future working life may be at stake

Systemic causes
- Endocrine diseases—diabetes, myxoedema, hyperthyroidism
- Metabolic diseases—hepatic failure, chronic renal failure
- Haematological—polycythaemia, iron deficiency anaemia
- Malignancy—lymphoma, reticulosis, carcinomatosis
- Psychological—anxiety, parasitophobia
- Tropical infection—filariasis, hookworm
- Drugs—alkaloids

Investigations
- Skin scrapings for mycology
- Patch testing for allergies
- Full blood count, erythrocyte sedimentation rate, liver and renal function tests
- Urine analysis
- Stools for blood and parasites

In *herpes zoster* there may be a variable degree of itching, but this is overshadowed by the pain and discomfort of the fully developed lesions.

By contrast, *bullous impetigo* causes few symptoms, although there may be extensive blisters. Itching is usually not present.

Dermatitis herpetiformis is characterised by intense persistent and severe itching that patients often describe as being unendurable. Usual measures such as topical steroids and antihistamines have little if any effect.

By contrast, the blisters of *pemphigoid* do not itch although the earlier inflamed lesions can be irritating.

Parasites. Fleas and mites cause pruritic papules in groups. The patient may not realise that they may have been acquired after a walk in the country or encountering a dog or cat. *Nodular prurigo* may develop after insect bites and is characterised by persistent itching, lichenified papules, and nodules over the trunk and limbs. The patient attacks them vigorously and promotes a persisting "itch–scratch–itch" cycle which is very difficult to break.

Parasitophobia is characterised by the patient reporting the presence of small insects burrowing into the skin which persists despite all forms of treatment. The patient will produce small flakes of skin, fibres of clothing, and pieces of dust, usually in carefully folded pieces of paper, for examination. These should always be examined and the patient gently informed that no insect could be found but this will not be believed. Treatment is therefore very difficult and sometimes recourse has to be had to psychotropic drugs (see page 106).

Infestations with lice cause irritation and a scabies mite can cause widespread persistent pruritus, even though only a dozen or so active scabies burrows are present. It is always acquired by close human contact and the diagnosis may be missed unless an adequate history of personal contacts and a thorough clinical examination is carried out. However, a speculative diagnosis of scabies should be avoided.

Itching with no skin lesions

If no dermatological lesions are present generalised pruritus or itchy skin may indicate an underlying internal cause. In elderly patients, however, the skin may itch simply because it is dry. Hodgkin's disease may present with pruritus as a sign of the internal malignancy long before any other manifestations. A 35 year old ambulance driver attended the dermatology clinic with intense itching but a normal skin and no history of skin disease. His general health was good and both physical examination and all blood tests were normal. However, a chest *x* ray examination showed a mediastinal shadow that was found to be due to Hodgkin's lymphoma. Fortunately this was easily treated. Other forms of carcinoma rarely cause pruritus.

Metabolic and endocrine disease

Biliary obstruction and *chronic renal disease* cause intense pruritus. *Thyroid disease* can be associated with an itching skin. In hyperthyroidism the skin seems normal but in hypothyroidism there is dryness of the skin causing pruritus.

Blood diseases. Polycythaemia and iron deficiency are sometimes associated with itching skin.

Treatment

Treatment of the cause must be carried out when possible. Calamine lotion cools the skin with 0·5% menthol or 1% phenol in aqueous cream. Camphor-containing preparations and crotamiton (Eurax) are also helpful. Topical steroid ointments and occlusive dressings may help to prevent scratching and may help to break the itch–scratch–itch cycle. Emollients should be used for dry skin.

Topical local anaesthetics may give relief but intolerance develops and they can cause allergic reactions. Sedative antihistamines at night may be helpful. In liver failure cholestyramine powder may help to relieve the intense pruritus, as this is thought to be due to bile salts in the skin.

Antihistamines can be helpful both for their antipruritic effect and because many are sedative and enable the itching patient to sleep.

Pruritus ani is a common troublesome condition and the following points may be helpful:

- Advise gentle cleaning once daily and patients should be advised to avoid excessive washing.
- Avoid harsh toilet paper, especially if coloured, because cheap dyes irritate and cause allergies. Olive oil and cotton wool can be used instead.
- Weak topical steroids will help to reduce inflammation, with zinc cream or ointment as a protective layer on top.
- Anal leakage from an incompetent sphincter, skin tags, or haemorrhoids may require surgical treatment.
- There may be an anxiety or depression and prutitus ani itself can lead to irritability and depression.

Pruritus vulvae is a persistent irritation of the vulva which can be most distressing and is most common in postmenopausal women. It is important to eliminate any factors that may be preventing resolution. These include:

- Secondary infection with pyogenic bacteria or yeasts
- Eczema or contact dermatitis
- Lichen sclerosus atrophicus.

The adjacent vaginal mucosa should be examined to exclude an intraepithelial neoplasm or lichen planus. Treatment includes suitable antiseptic preparations such as 2% eosin, regular but not excessive washing, emollients, and topical steroids, bearing in mind the possibility of infection.

Further reading

Adams RM. *Occupational skin disease*, 2nd ed. Philadelphia: Saunders, 1990

Arndt KA. *Manual of dermatological therapeutics*, 5th ed. New York: Little, 1995

Atherton DJ. *Eczema in childhood. The facts.* Oxford: Oxford University Press, 1994

Cronin E. *Contact dermatitis.* Edinburgh: Churchill Livingstone, 1980

Fisher AA. *Contact dermatitis*, 3rd ed. Baltimore: Williams and Wilkins, 1986

Foussereau J, Benezra JE, Maibach H. *Occupational contact dermatitis.* Copenhagen: Munksgaard, 1982

Schwanitz HJ. *Atopic palmoplantar eczema.* Berlin: Springer-Verlag, 1988

5 Treatment of eczema and inflammatory dermatoses

Treat the patient, not just the rash. Many patients accept their skin condition with equanimity but others suffer much distress, especially if the face and hands are affected. Acceptance by the doctor of the individual and his or her attitudes to the disease goes a long way to helping the patient live with the condition.

The common inflammatory skin diseases can nearly always be improved or cleared, but it is wise not to promise a permanent cure.

Be realistic about the treatment people can apply in their own homes. It is easy to unthinkingly give patients with a widespread rash a large amount of ointment to apply twice daily, which is hardly used because: (a) they have a busy job or young children and simply do not have time to apply ointment to the whole skin; (b) they have arthritic or other limitations of movement and can reach only a small part of the body; (c) the tar or other ointment is smelly or discolours their clothes. Most of us have been guilty of forgetting these factors at one time or another.

Dry skin tends to be itchy, so advise minimal use of soap. Emollients are used to soften the skin, and the simpler the better. Emulsifying ointment BP is cheap and effective but rather thick. By mixing two tablespoons in a kitchen blender with a pint of water, the result is a creamy mixture that can easily be used in the bath. A useful preparation is equal parts of white soft paraffin and liquid paraffin. Various proprietary bath oils are available and can be applied directly to wet skin. There are many proprietary emollients.

Wet weeping lesions should generally be treated with creams rather than ointments (which remain on the surface).

Steroid ointments are effective in relieving inflammation and itching but are not always used effectively. Advise patients to use a strong steroid (such as betamethasone or fluocinolone acetonide) frequently for a few days to bring the condition under control; then change to a weaker steroid (dilute betamethasone, fluocinolone, clobetasone, hydrocortisone) less frequently. Strong steroids should not be continued for long periods, and, as a rule, do not prescribe any steroid stronger than hydrocortisone for the face. Strong steroids can cause atrophy of the skin if used for long periods, particularly when applied under occlusive dressings. On the face they may lead to florid telangiectasia and acne-like pustules. Avoid using steroids on ulcerated areas. Prolonged use of topical steroids may mask an underlying bacterial or fungal infection.

Immunosuppressants are a valuable adjunct in severe cases not responding to topical treatment and antibiotics. Ciclosporin is usually given on an intermittent basis, with careful monitoring for side effects. Azathioprine is also used, provided the thiopurine methyl transferase (TPMT) level is normal.

Tacrolimus is an immunosuppressant that has recently become available in two strengths as an ointment. It promises to be a successful treatment but is relatively expensive.

Specific treatment

Wet, inflamed, exuding lesions
(1) Use wet soaks with plain water, normal saline, or aluminium acetate (0·6%). Potassium permanganate (0·1%) solution should be used if there is any sign of infection.

Treatment guidelines
- Treat the patient, not just the rash
- Complete cure may not be possible
- Be realistic about the problems of applying treatments at home
- Make sure the patient understands how to carry out the treatment
- Advise using emollients and minimal soap
- Provide detailed guidance on using steroids

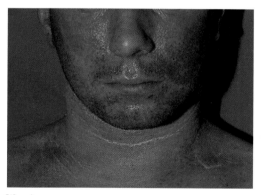
Weeping eczema

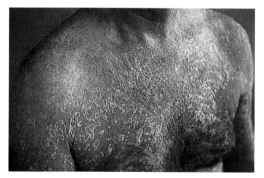
Acute erythema

(2) Use wet compresses rather than dry dressings ("wet wraps").
(3) Steroid *creams* should be used as outlined above. Greasy ointment bases tend to float off on the exudate.
(4) A combined steroid–antibiotic cream is often needed as infection readily develops.
(5) Systemic antibiotics may be required in severe cases. Take swabs for bacteriological examination first.

Dry, scaling, lichenified lesions
(1) Use emollients.
(2) Use steroid *ointments*, with antibiotics if infection is present.
(3) A weak coal tar preparation or ichthammol can be used on top of the ointments. This is particularly useful at night to prevent itching. 1–2% coal tar can be prescribed in an ointment. For hard, lichenified skin salicylic acid can be incorporated and the following formulation has been found useful in our department:
  (a) Coal tar solution BP 10%, salicylic acid 2%, and unguentum drench to 100%.
  (b) 1% ichthammol and 15% zinc oxide in white soft paraffin is less likely to irritate than tar and is suitable for children.
(4) In treating psoriasis start with a weaker tar preparation and progress to a stronger one.
(5) For thick, hyperkeratotic lesions, particularly in the scalp, salicylic acid is useful. It can be prescribed as 2–5% in aqueous cream, 1–2% in arachis oil, or 6% gel.

It is often easiest for the patient to apply the preparation to the scalp at night and wash it out the next morning with a tar shampoo.

Infection
Remember that secondary infection may be a cause of persisting lesions.

Hand dermatitis
Hand dermatitis poses a particular problem in management and it is important that protection is continued after the initial rash has healed because it takes some time for the skin to recover its barrier function. Ointments or creams should be reapplied each time the hands have been washed.

It is useful to give patients a list of simple instructions such as those shown in the box on the right.

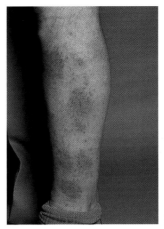

Lichenified eczema

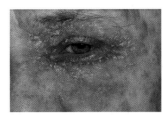

Infected eczema

Hand dermatitis: hints on management
- Hand washing: use tepid water and soap without perfume or colouring or chemicals added; dry carefully, especially between fingers
- When in wet work: wear cotton gloves under rubber gloves (or plastic if you are allergic to rubber); try not to use hot water and cut down to 15 minutes at a time if possible; remove rings before wet or dry work; use running water if possible
- Wear gloves in cold weather and for dusty work
- Use only ointments prescribed for you
- Things to avoid on unprotected skin:
  Shampoo
  Peeling fruits and vegetables, especially citrus fruits
  Polishes of all kinds
  Solvents, for example, white spirit, thinners, turpentine
  Hair lotions, creams, and dyes
  Detergents and strong cleansing agents
  "Unknown" chemicals
- Use "moisturisers" or emollients which have been recommended by your doctor to counteract dryness

Further reading
Atherton DJ. *Diet and children with eczema*. London: National Eczema Society, 1986
Launer JM. *A practical guide to the management of eczema for general practitioners*. London: National Eczema Society, 1988
Mackie RM. *Eczema and dermatitis*. London: Martin Dunitz, 1983
Orton C. *Eczema relief: a complete guide to all remedies—alternative and orthodox*. London: Thorsons, 1990

6   Rashes with epidermal changes

Familiarity with the clinical features of psoriasis and eczema, which all clinicians see from time to time, provides a basis for comparison with other rather less common conditions. The characteristics that each condition has in common with psoriasis and eczema are highlighted in the relevant tables.

Lichen planus

Like psoriasis, the lesions are well defined and raised. They also occur in areas of trauma—the Koebner's phenomenon. There is no constant relation to stress.

Unlike psoriasis, there is no family history. Itching is common. The distribution is on the flexor aspects of the limbs, particularly the ankles and wrists, rather than on the extensor surfaces, as in psoriasis. It also occurs on the trunk. However, localised forms of lichen planus can occur on the shin, palm, and soles or elsewhere.

Nail involvement is less common than in psoriasis. There may be thinning and atrophy of part or all of a nail and these often take the form of a longitudinal groove, sometimes with destruction of the nail plate. The oral mucosa is commonly affected with a white, net-like appearance and sometimes ulceration.

The typical flat topped lesions have a shiny hyperkeratotic lichenified surface with a violaceous colour, interrupted by milky white streaks—Wickham's striae.

Less commonly, very thick hypertrophic lesions occur and also follicular lesions. Lichen planus is one cause of localised alopecia on the scalp as a result of hair follicle destruction.

Lichen planus usually resolves over many months to leave residual brown or grey macules. In the oral mucosa and areas subject to trauma ulceration can occur.

Characteristics of lichen planus

Clinical features of psoriasis	Clinical features of eczema
Possible family history	Possible family history
Sometimes related to stress	Sometimes worse with stress
Itching—rare	Usually itching
Extensor surfaces and trunk	Flexor surfaces and face
Well defined, raised lesions	Poorly demarcated lesions
Hyperkeratosis	Oedema, vesicles, lichenification
Scaling, bleeding points beneath scales	Secondary infection sometimes present
Koebner's phenomenon	
Nails affected	
Scalp affected	
Mucous membranes not affected	

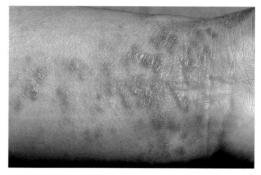

Lichen planus—wrist

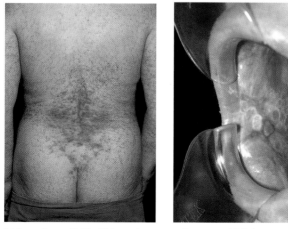

Lichen planus (left). Lichen planus—oral mucosa (right)

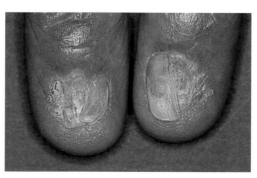

Lichen planus—nails

Treatment

There is usually a gradual response to topical steroids, but in very extensive and inflamed lesions systemic steroids may be needed. Localised hypertrophic lesions can be treated with intralesional injections.

Similar rashes

Lichenified eczema

This is also itchy and may occur on the ankles and wrists. The edge of the lesion is less well defined and is irregular. The flat topped, shiny papules are absent.

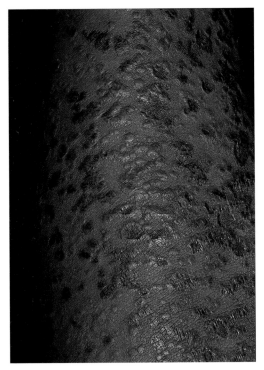

Lichen planus

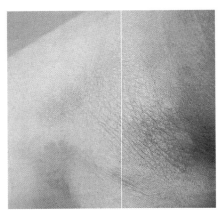

Lichenified eczema

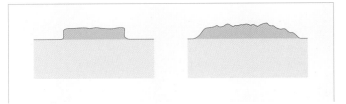

Guttate psoriasis—section through lesion (left); lichenified eczema—section through lesion (right)

Guttate psoriasis

Guttate psoriasis is not as itchy as lichen planus. Scaling erythematous lesions do not have the lichenified surface of lichen planus.

Pityriasis lichenoides

The lesions have a mica-like scale overlying an erythematous papule.

Drug eruptions

Rashes with many features of lichen planus can occur in patients taking:

- Chloroquine
- Chlorpropamide   The three "C"s
- Chlorothiazide
- Anti-inflammatory drugs
- Gold preparations

It also occurs in those handling colour developers.

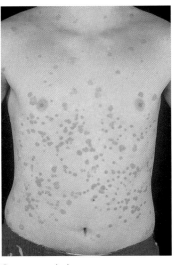

Guttate psoriasis

Lichen planus

- Flexor surfaces
- Mucous membranes affected
- Itching common
- Violaceous colour
- Wickham's striae
- Small discrete lesions
- Lichenified

Treatment

The main symptom of itching is relieved to some extent by moderately potent steroid ointments. Very hypertrophic lesions may respond to strong steroid preparations under polythene occlusion. Careful intralesional injections may be effective in persistent lesions. In very extensive, severe lichen planus systemic steroids may be indicated.

Pathology of lichen planus

As expected from the clinical appearance, there is hypertrophy and thickening of the epidermis with increased keratin. The white streaks seen clinically occur where there is pronounced thickness of the granular layer and underlying infiltrate. Degenerating basal cells may form "colloid bodies". The basal layer is being eaten away by an aggressive band of lymphocytes, the remaining papillae having a "saw toothed" appearance.

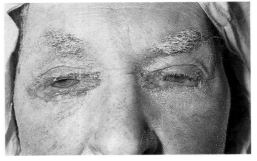

Lichen planus—pathology

Seborrhoeic dermatitis

Seborrhoeic dermatitis has nothing to do with sebum or any other kind of greasiness. There are two distinct types, adult and infantile.

Adult seborrhoeic dermatitis

The adult type is more common in men and in those with a tendency to scaling and dandruff in the scalp. There are several commonly affected areas:

- Seborrhoeic dermatitis affects the central part of the face, scalp, ears, and eyebrows. There may be an associated blepharitis, giving some red eyes and also otitis externa.
- The lesions over the sternum sometimes start as a single "medallion" lesion. A flower-like "petaloid" pattern can occur. The back may be affected as well.
- Lesions also occur in well defined areas in the axillae and groin and beneath the breasts.

Typically the lesions are discrete and erythematous and they may develop a yellow crust. The lesions tend to develop from the hair follicles. It is a persistent condition that varies in severity.

Clinically and pathologically the condition has features of both psoriasis and eczema. There is thickening of the epidermis with some of the inflammatory changes of psoriasis and the intercellular oedema of eczema. Parakeratosis—the presence of nuclei above the basement layer—may be noticeable. Recently, increased numbers of *Pityrosporum ovale* organisms have been reported.

Treatment

Topical steroids produce a rapid improvement, but not permanent clearing. Topical preparations containing salicylic acid, sulphur, or ichthammol may help in long term control. Triazole antifungal drugs by mouth have been reported to produce clearing and can be used topically. These drugs clear yeasts and fungi from the skin, including *P. ovale*, which is further evidence for the role of this organism.

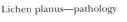

Seborrhoeic dermatitis

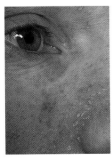

Seborrhoeic dermatitis affecting centre of face

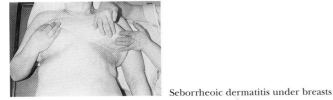

Seborrhoeic dermatitis under breasts

Characteristics of seborrhoeic dermatitis

Clinical features of psoriasis	Clinical features of eczema
Possible family history	Possible family history
Sometimes related to stress	Sometimes worse with stress
Itching—rare	Usually itching
Extensor surfaces and trunk	Flexor surfaces and face
Well defined, raised lesions	Poorly, demarcated lesions
Hyperkeratosis	Oedema, vesicles, lichenification
Scaling, bleeding points beneath scales	Secondary infection sometimes, present
Koebner's phenomenon	
Nails affected	
Scalp affected	
Mucous membranes not affected	

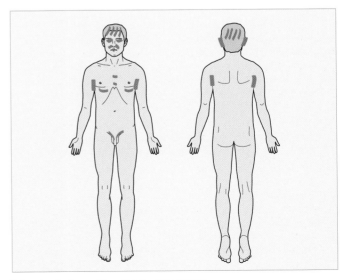

Seborrhoeic dermatitis—distribution pattern

29

Infantile seborrhoeic dermatitis

In infants less than six months old a florid red eruption occurs with well defined lesions on the trunk and confluent areas in the flexures associated with scaling of the scalp. There is no consistent association with the adult type of seborrhoeic dermatitis. It has been suggested that infantile seborrhoeic dermatitis is a variant of atopic eczema. It is said to be more common in bottle fed infants. A high proportion of affected infants develop atopic eczema later but there are distinct differences.

Itching is present in atopic eczema but not in seborrhoeic dermatitis.

The *clinical course* of atopic eczema is prolonged with frequent exacerbation, whereas seborrhoeic dermatitis clears in a few weeks and seldom recurs.

Treatment comprises emollients, avoiding soap, and applying hydrocortisone combined with an antibiotic plus nystatin (for example, Terra-Cortril plus nystatin cream). Hydrocortisone can be used on the scalp.

Allergy

IgE concentrations are often raised in atopic eczema and food allergy is common, but not in seborrhoeic dermatitis.

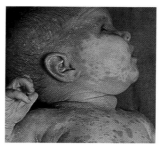
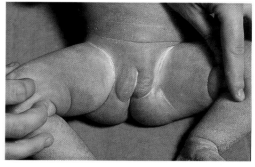

Infantile Seborrhoeic dermatitis

Perioral dermatitis

Perioral dermatitis is possibly a variant of seborrhoeic dermatitis, with some features of acne. Papules and pustules develop around the mouth and chin. It occurs mainly in women.

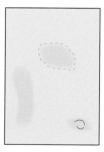

Perioral dermatitis

Pityriasis rosea

The word "pityriasis" is from the Greek for bran, and the fine bran-like scales on the surface are a characteristic feature. The numerous pale pink oval or round patches can be confused with psoriasis or discoid eczema. The history helps because this condition develops as an acute eruption and the patient can often point to a simple initial lesion—the herald patch.

There is commonly slight itching. Pityriasis rosea occurs mainly in the second and third decade, often during the winter months. "Clusters" of cases occur but not true epidemics. This suggests an infective basis. There may be prodromal symptoms with malaise, fever, or lymphadenopathy. Numerous causes have been suggested, from allergy to fungi; the current favourite is a virus infection.

The typical patient is an adolescent or young adult, who is often more than a little concerned about the sudden appearance of a widespread rash. The lesions are widely distributed, often following skin creases, and concentrated on the trunk with scattered lesions on the limbs. The face and scalp may be affected.

Early lesions are red with fine scales—usually 1–4 cm in diameter. The initial herald patch is larger and may be confused with a fungal infection. Subsequently the widespread eruption develops in a matter of days or, rarely, weeks. As time goes by the lesions clear to give a slight pigmentation with a collarette of scales facing towards the centre.

Similar rashes

Discoid eczema presents with itching and lesions with erythema, oedema, and crusting rather than scaling. Vesicles may be present. The rash persists unchanged.

A *drug eruption* can sometimes produce similar lesions.

In *guttate psoriasis* the lesions are more sharply defined and smaller (0·5–1·0 cm) and have waxy scales.

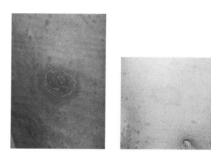
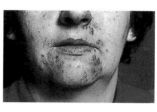

Pityriasis rosea—herald lesions

Characteristics of pityriasis rosea

Clinical features of psoriasis	Clinical features of eczema
Possible family history	Possible family history
Sometimes related to stress	Sometimes worse with stress
Itching—rare	Usually itching
Extensor surfaces and trunk	Flexor surfaces and face
Well defined, raised lesions	Poorly demarcated lesions
Hyperkeratosis	Oedema, vesicles, lichenification
Scaling, bleeding points beneath scales	Secondary infection sometimes present
Köebner's phenomenon	
Nails affected	
Scalp affected	
Mucous membranes not affected	

Pathology

Histological changes are non-specific, showing slight inflammatory changes in the dermis, oedema, and slight hyperkeratosis.

Pityriasis lichenoides

Pityriasis lichenoides is a less common condition occurring in acute and chronic forms.

The *acute* form presents with widespread pink papules which itch and form crusts, sometimes with vesicle formation suggestive of chickenpox. There may be ulceration. The lesions may develop in crops and resolve over a matter of weeks.

The *chronic* form presents as reddish brown papules—often with a "mica"-like scale that reveals a smooth, red surface underneath, unlike the bleeding points of psoriasis. In lichen planus there is no superficial scale and blistering is unusual.

The distribution is over the trunk, thighs, and arms, usually sparing the face and scalp.

The underlying pathology—vascular dilatation and a lymphocytic infiltrate with a keratotic scale—is in keeping with the clinical appearance. The cause is unknown.

Treatment is with topical steroids. Ultraviolet light treatment is also helpful.

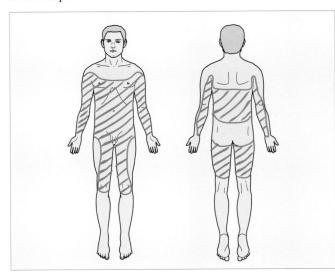

Pityriasis lichenoides—distribution pattern

Pityriasis versicolor

Pityriasis versicolor is a skin eruption that usually develops after sun exposure with white macules on the tanned skin but pale brown patches on the covered areas, hence the name versicolor, or variable colour. The lesions are: (a) flat; (b) only partially depigmented—areas of vitiligo are totally white; and (c) do not show inflammation or vesicles.

The causative organism is a yeast, *Pityrosporum orbiculare*, that takes advantage of some unknown change in the epidermis and develops a proliferative, stubby, mycelial form, *Malassezia furfur*. This otherwise incidental information can be simply put to practical use by taking a superficial scraping from a lesion on to a microscope slide—add a drop of potassium hydroxide or water with a coverslip. The organisms are readily seen under the microscope as spherical yeast forms and mycelial rods, resembling "grapes and bananas" ("spaghetti and meatballs" in the United States).

Treatment is simple: selenium sulphide shampoo applied regularly with ample water while showering or bathing will clear the infection. The colour change may take some time to clear.

Characteristics of pityriasis lichenoides

Clinical features of psoriasis	Clinical features of eczema
Possible family history	Possible family history
Sometimes related to stress	Sometimes worse with stress
Itching—rare	Usually itching
Extensor surfaces and trunk	Flexor surfaces and face
Well defined, raised lesions	Poorly demarcated lesions
Hyperkeratosis	Oedema, vesicles, lichenification
Scaling, bleeding points beneath scales	Secondary infection sometimes present
Koebner's phenomenon	
Nails affected	
Scalp affected	
Mucous membranes not affected	

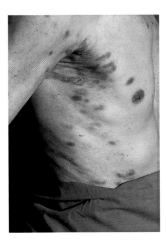

Pityriasis lichenoides showing acute erythematous rash

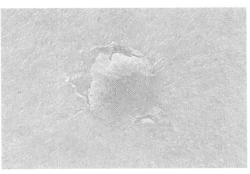

A mica scale pityriasis lichenoides

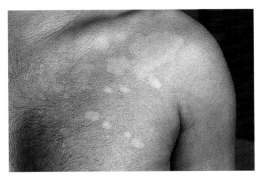

Pityriasis versicolor skin lesions

Ketoconazole shampoo is an effective alternative. Oral terbinafine, which is very effective in other fungal infections, has no effect.

Desquamating stage of generalised erythema

Any extensive acute erythema, from the erythroderma of psoriasis to a penicillin rash, commonly shows a stage of shedding large flakes of skin—desquamation—as it resolves. If only this stage is seen it can be confused with psoriasis.

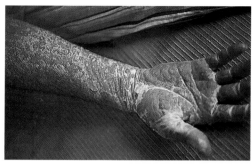

Desquamation

Localised lesions with epidermal changes

Psoriasis, seborrhoeic dermatitis, atopic eczema, and contact dermatitis can all present with localised lesions.

Psoriasis may affect only the flexures, occur as a genital lesion, or affect only the palms. The lack of itching and epidermal changes with a sharp edge help in differentiation from infective or infiltrative lesions.

Seborrhoeic dermatitis can occur in the axillae or scalp with no lesions of other areas.

In *atopic eczema* the "classical" sites in children—flexures of the elbows and knees and the face—may be modified in adults to localised vesicular lesions on the hands and feet in older patients. Some atopic adults develop severe, persistent generalised eczematous changes.

Contact dermatitis is usually localised, by definition, to the areas in contact with irritant or allergen. Wide areas can be affected in reactions to clothing or washing powder, and sometimes the reaction extends beyond the site of contact.

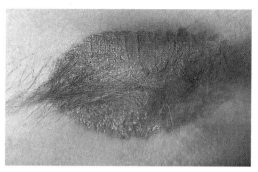

Flexural seborrhoeic dermatitis

Fungal infections

Apart from athlete's foot, toenail infections, and tinea cruris (most commonly in men), "ringworm" is in fact not as common as is supposed. The damp, soggy, itching skin of athlete's foot is well known. An itching, red diffuse rash in the groin differentiates tinea cruris from psoriasis. However, erythrasma, a bacterial infection, may be confused with seborrhoeic dermatitis and psoriasis—skin scrapings can be taken for culture of *Corynebacterium minutissimum* or, more simply, coral pink fluorescence shown with Wood's light. The scaling macules from dog and cat ringworm (*Microsporum canis*) itch greatly, whereas the indurated pustular, boggy lesion (kerion) of cattle ringworm is quite distinctive.

Fungal infection of the axillae is rare; a red rash here is more likely to be due to erythrasma or seborrhoeic dermatitis.

Tinea cruris is very unusual before puberty and is uncommon in women.

In all cases of suspected fungal infection skin scrapings should be taken on to black paper, in which they can be folded and sent to the laboratory. Special "kits" are available, which contain folded black paper and Sellotape strips on slides for taking a superficial layer of epidermis.

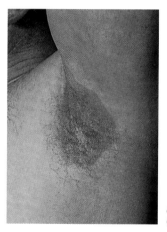

Corynebacterium minutissimum (erythrasma)

Lupus erythematosus

There are two forms of this condition: discoid, which is usually limited to the skin, and systemic, in which the skin lesions are associated with renal disease, arthritis, and other disorders. There is also a subacute type with limited systemic involvement.

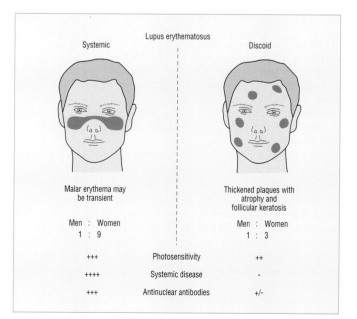

	Lupus erythematosus	
Systemic		Discoid
Malar erythema may be transient		Thickened plaques with atrophy and follicular keratosis
Men : Women 1 : 9		Men : Women 1 : 3
+++	Photosensitivity	++
++++	Systemic disease	-
+++	Antinuclear antibodies	+/-

Characteristics of systemic and discoid lupus erythematosus

Systemic lupus erythematosus, which is much more common in women than men, can be an acute, fulminating, multisystem disease that requires intensive treatment, or a more chronic progressive illness. Characteristically there is malar erythema with marked photosensitivity and a butterfly pattern. It may be transient. There may be scalp involvement as well with alopecia and also telangiectasia of the perifungal blood vessels. Mouth ulcers may also be present. Systemic involvement may cause nephritis, polyarteritis, leukopenia, pleurisy, myocarditis, and central nervous system involvement.

Systemic lupus erythematosus can present in many forms and imitate other diseases. The facial rash can resemble rosacea, cosmetic allergy, or sun sensitivity. Systemic involvement may present with lassitude, weight loss, anaemia, arthritis, renal failure, dyspnoea, or cardiac signs among others.

Criteria for making a diagnosis of systemic lupus erythematosus have been established, of which at least four must be present.

In the subacute variety there is less severe systemic involvement, with scattered lesions occurring on the face, scalp, chest, and arms.

Treatment is with systemic steroids, with immunosuppressive agents if necessary. Antimalarial drugs, such as hydroxychloroquine, are more effective in the subacute type.

In discoid lupus erythematosus there are well defined lesions with a combination of atrophy and hyperkeratosis of the hair follicles giving a "nutmeg grater" appearance. They occur predominantly on the cheeks, nose, and forehead. It is about three times as common in women as men, which is a lower ratio than in the systemic variety. There is a tendency for the skin lesions to gradually progress and to flare up on sun exposure. It is rare for progression to the systemic type to occur.

Treatment is with moderate to very potent topical steroids and hydroxychloroquine by mouth, together with suitable sun screens.

Fixed drug eruptions

Generalised drug eruptions are considered under erythema, but there is a localised form recurring every time the drug is used. There is usually a well defined, erythematous plaque, sometimes with vesicles. Crusting, scaling, and pigmentation occur as the lesion heals. It is usually found on the limbs, and more than one lesion can occur.

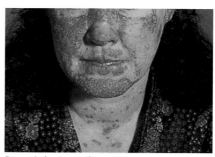

Systemic lupus erythematosus—subacute

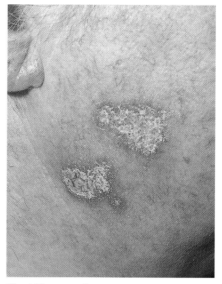

Discoid lupus erythematosus

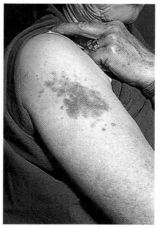

Fixed drug eruption

Criteria for diagnosing systemic lupus erythematosus

- Malar rash
- Discoid plaques
- Photosensitivity
- Mouth ulcers
- Arthritis
- Serositis
- Renal disease
- Neurological disease
- Haematological changes
- Immunological changes
- Antinuclear antibodies

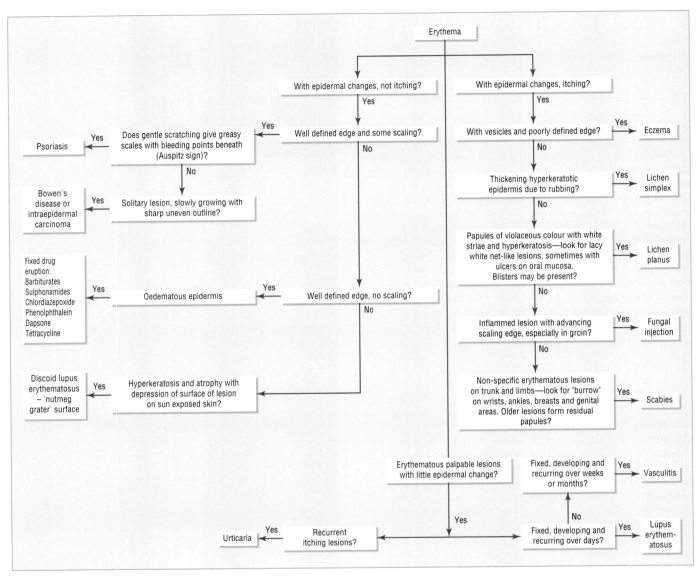

Causes of epidermal rashes

7 Rashes arising in the dermis

The erythemas

Complex reactions occurring in the capillaries and arterioles of the skin cause erythema, which is simply redness of the skin. This may present as flat macules or as papules, which are raised above the surrounding skin. The lesions may be transient or last for weeks, constant or variable in distribution, with or without vesicles.

It is possible to recognise specific patterns within this plethora of clinical signs, but even the most experienced dermatologist may be reduced to making a general diagnosis of "toxic" erythema. The best we can do therefore is to recognise the common types of erythema and list the possible causes. It is then a matter of deciding on the most likely underlying condition or group of conditions—for example, bacterial infection or autoimmune systemic disease.

Morphology and distribution
Because there can be the same cause for a variety of erythematous rashes detailed descriptions are of limited use. None the less, there are some characteristic patterns.

Morbilliform
The presentation of measles is well known, with the appearance of Koplik's spots on the mucosa, photophobia with conjunctivitis, and red macules behind the ears, spreading to the face, trunk, and limbs. The prodromal symptoms and conjunctivitis are absent in drug eruptions. Other viral conditions, including those caused by echoviruses, rubella, infectious mononucleosis, and erythema infectiosum, may have to be considered.

Scarlatiniform
These rashes are similar to that in scarlet fever, when an acute erythematous eruption occurs in relation to a streptococcal infection. Characteristically erythema is widespread on the trunk. There is intense erythema and engorgement of the pharyngeal lymphoid tissue with an exudate and a "strawberry" tongue. Bacterial infections can produce a similar rash, as can drug rashes, without the systemic symptoms.

Figurate erythemas
These are chronic erythematous rashes forming annular or serpiginous patterns. There may be underlying malignancy or connective tissue disease.

Erythema multiforme
Erythema multiforme is sometimes misdiagnosed because of the variety of lesions and number of possible precipitating causes; some of these are listed in the box on the right.

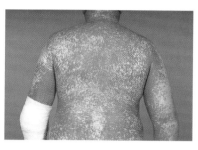

Erythema from antibiotics

Causes of "toxic" erythema

Drugs
- Antibiotics, barbiturates, thiazides

Infections
- Any recent infections such as streptococcal throat infection or erysipelas; spirochaetal infections; viral infections

Systemic causes
- Pregnancy; connective tissue disease; malignancy

Erythema multiforme: precipitating causes

Infections
- Herpes simplex—the commonest cause
- Mycoplasma infection
- Infectious mononucleosis
- Poliomyelitis (vaccine)
- Many other viral and bacterial infections
- Any focal sepsis
- BCG inoculaton

Collagen disease
- Systemic lupus erythematosus
- Polyarteritis nodosa

Neoplasia
- Hodgkin's disease
- Myeloma
- Carcinoma

Chronic inflammation
- Sarcoidosis
- Wegener's granuloma

Drugs
- Barbiturates
- Sulphonamides
- Penicillin
- Phenothiazine and many others

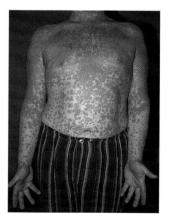

Erythema multiforme

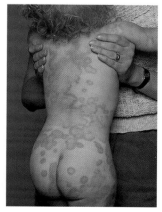

Erythema multiforme

Clinical picture

The usual erythematous lesions occur in crops on the limbs and trunk. Each lesion may extend, leaving a cyanotic centre, which produces an "iris" or "target" lesion. Bullae may develop in the lesions and on the mucous membranes. A severe bullous form, with lesions on the mucous membranes, is known as the Stevens–Johnson syndrome. There may be neural and bronchial changes as well. Barbiturates, sulphonamides, and other drugs, are the most common cause.

Histologically there are inflammatory changes, vasodilatation, and degeneration of the epidermis.

A condition that may be confused is Sweet's syndrome, which presents as acute plum coloured raised painful lesions on the limbs—sometimes the face and neck—with fever. It is more common in women. The alternative name, "acute febrile neutrophilic dermatosis", describes the presentation and the pathological findings of a florid neutrophilic infiltrate. There is often a preceding upper respiratory infection. Treatment with steroids produces a rapid response but recurrences are common.

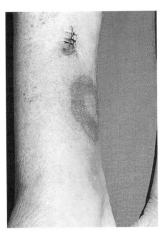
Annular lesions of erythema multiforme

Erythema induratum

Erythema induraturn occurs on the lower legs posteriorly, usually in women, with diffuse, indurated dusky red lesions that may ulcerate. It is more common in patients with poor cutaneous circulation. Epithelioid cell granulomas may form.

This erythema was originally described in association with tuberculous infection elsewhere in the body (Bazin's disease). It represents a vasculitic reaction to the infection, and when there is no tuberculous infection another chronic infection may be responsible.

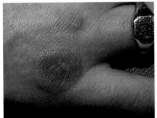
Annular lesions of erythema multiforme

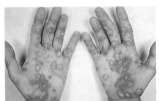
Blistering lesions of erythema multiforme

Erythema nodosum

Erythema nodosum occurs as firm, gradually developing lesions, predominantly on the extensor aspect of the legs. They are tender and progress over four to eight weeks from an acute erythematous stage to residual lesions resembling bruises.

Single or multiple lesions occur, varying in size from 1 to 5 cm. The lesions are often preceded by an upper respiratory tract infection and may be associated with fever and arthralgia. Infections (streptococcal, tuberculous, viral, and fungal) and sarcoidosis are the commonest underlying conditions. Drugs can precipitate erythema nodosum, the contraceptive pill and the sulphonamides being the commonest cause. Ulcerative colitis, Crohn's disease, and lymphoma may also be associated with the condition.

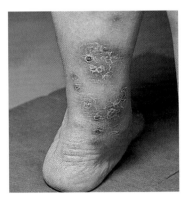
Erythema induratum

Rashes due to drugs

There is an almost infinite variety of types of drug reaction.

External contact with drugs can cause a contact dermatitis presenting with eczematous changes. This occurs commonly with neomycin and bacitracin. Chloramphenicol and sulphonamides from ophthalmic preparations can also cause dermatitis around the eyes. Penicillin is a potent sensitiser so is not used for topical treatment.

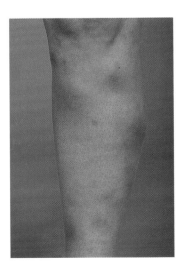
Erythema nodosum

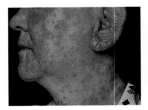
Topical neomycin allergy

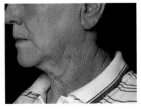
Same patient after withdrawing neomycin

Drugs used systemically can cause a localised fixed drug eruption or a more diffuse macular or papular erythema, symmetrically distributed. In the later stages exfoliation, with shedding scales of skin, may develop. Antibiotics, particularly penicillins, are the most common cause. They also cause erythema multiforme as already mentioned.

Penicillins are the most common cause of drug rashes, which range from acute anaphylaxis to persistent diffuse erythematous lesions. Joint pains, fever, and proteinuria may be associated, as in serum sickness.

Ampicillin often produces a characteristic erythematous maculopapular rash on the limbs seven to 20 days after the start of treatment. Such rashes occur in nearly all patients with infectious mononucleosis who are given ampicillin.

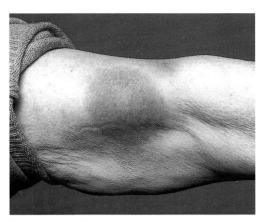

Fixed drug eruption

Vasculitis

Inflammation associated with immune complexes in the capillaries and small blood vessels is part of the pathological changes of many of the conditions described above. The term vasculitis is also used clinically to describe a variable clinical picture with red macules and papules and with necrosis and bruising in severe cases. In children purpura is more prominent and these cases are classified as Henoch–Schönlein purpura. The legs and arms are usually affected. Skin signs are preceded by malaise and fever with arthropathy and there may be associated urticaria. As a high proportion of cases are associated with systemic lesions, it is essential to check for renal, skeletal, gastrointestinal, and central nervous system disease. In children with Henoch–Schönlein purpura nephritis is common.

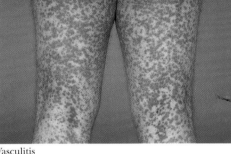

Vasculitis

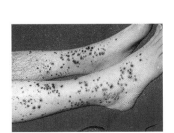

Acute vasculitis with necrosis

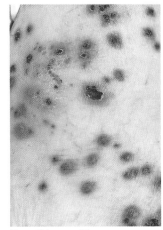

Necrotising angiitis

Drug reactions

Blistering eruptions
- Barbiturates
- Sulphonamides
- Iodines or bromides
- Chlorpropamide
- Salicylates
- Phenylbutazone

Lichen planus like reactions
- Chloroquine
- Chlorothiazide
- Chlorpropamide

Photosensitivity (seen on areas exposed to light)
- Thiazide diuretics
- Sulphonamides
- Tetracyclines

Vasculitis
- Inflammation around dilated capillaries and small blood vessels
- A common component of the erythemas
- May occur as red macules and papules with necrotic lesions on the extremities
- In children a purpuric type (Henoch–Schönlein purpura) occurs in association with nephritis
- Systemic lesions may occur, with renal, joint, gastrointestinal, and central nervous system involvement

Purpura

Is seen on the skin as a result of:
- Thrombocytopenia—platelet deficiency
- Senile purpura—due to shearing of capillaries as a result of defective supporting connective tissue
- Purpura in patients on corticosteroid treatment—similar to senile purpura
- Schamberg's disease—brown macules and red spots resembling cayenne pepper on the legs of men
- Associated vasculitis

Some conditions associated with vasculitis
- Infection—streptococcal, hepatitis
- Drugs—numerous, including sulphonamides, penicillin, phenothiazine, phenacitin
- Chemicals—insecticides, weed killers, phenolic compounds
- Connective tissue diseases—systemic lupus erythematosus, rheumatoid arthritis
- Lymphoma and leukaemia
- Dysproteinaemias

Urticaria

In this condition itching red weals develop; they resemble the effects of stinging nettle (*Urtica dioica*) on the skin. The condition may be associated with allergic reactions, infection, or physical stimuli, but in most patients no cause can be found. Similar lesions may precede, or be associated with, vasculitis (urticarial vasculitis), pemphigoid, or dermatitis herpetiformis.

The histological changes may be very slight but usually there is oedema, vasodilatation, and a cellular infiltrate of lymphocytes, polymorphs, and histiocytes. Various vasoactive substances are thought to be involved, including histamine, kinins, leukotrienes, prostaglandins, and complement.

Angio-oedema is due to oedema of the subcutaneous tissues; it can occur rapidly and may involve the mucous membranes. Hereditary angio-oedema is a rare form with recurrent severe episodes of subcutaneous oedema, swelling of the mucous membranes, and systemic symptoms. Laryngeal oedema is the most serious complication.

The *physical urticarias*, which account for about 25% of cases, include dermatographism and the pressure, cold, heat, solar, cholinergic, and aquagenic urticarias.

Dermatographism is an exaggerated release of histamine from stroking the skin firmly with a hard object, such as the end of a pencil. *Pressure urticaria* is caused by sustained pressure from clothing, hard seats, and footwear; it may last some hours. *Cold urticaria* varies in severity and is induced by cold, particulary by cold winds or by the severe shock of bathing in cold water. It appears early in life—in infancy in the rare familial form. In a few cases abnormal serum proteins may be found. *Heat urticaria* is rare, but warm environments often make physical urticaria worse. *Solar urticaria* is a rare condition in which sunlight causes an acute urticarial eruption. Tolerance to sun exposure may develop in areas of the body normally exposed to sun. There is sensitivity to a wide spectrum of ultraviolet light. *Cholinergic urticaria* is characterised by the onset of itching urticarial papules after exertion, stress, or exposure to heat. The injection of cholinergic drugs induces similar lesions in some patients. *Aquagenic urticaria* occurs on contact with water, regardless of the temperature.

Non-physical urticaria may be acute in association with allergic reactions to insect bites, drugs, and other factors. Chronic recurrent urticaria is fairly common. Innumerable causes have been suggested but, to the frustration of patient and doctor alike, it is often impossible to identify any specific factor.

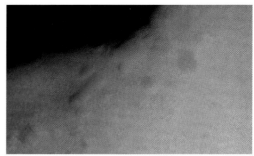

Urticaria

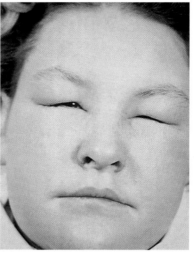

Angio-oedema

Some reported causes of non-physical urticaria

- Food allergies—fish, eggs, dairy products, chocolate, nuts, strawberries, pork, tomatoes
- Food additives—for example, tartrazine dyes, sodium benzoates
- Salicylates—both in medicines and foods
- Infection—bacterial, viral, and protozoal
- Systemic disorders—autoimmune and "collagen" diseases; reticuloses, carcinoma, and dysproteinaemias
- Contact urticaria—may occur from contact with meat, fish, vegetables, plants, and animals, among many other factors
- Papular urticaria—a term used for persistent itching papules at the site of insect bites; it is also sometimes applied to urticaria from other causes
- Inhalants—for example, house dust, animal danders

Treatment of urticaria

- Eliminate possible causative factors, such as aspirin, and by a diet free from food additives
- Antihistamines. Also, H_2 blockers, for example, cimetidine
- Adrenaline can be used for acute attacks, particularly if there is angio-oedema of the respiratory tract
- Systemic corticosteroids should not be used for chronic urticaria but may be needed for acute urticarial vasculitis

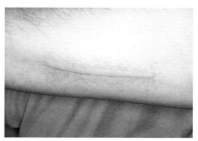

Dermatographism

Further reading

Berlit P, Moore P. *Vasculitis, rheumatic diseases and the nervous system.* Berlin: Springer-Verlag, 1992

Champion RH, Greaves MW, Black AK. *The urticarias.* Edinburgh: Churchill Livingstone, 1985

Czametzki BM. *Urticaria.* Berlin: Springer-Verlag, 1986

8 Blisters and pustules

Development, duration, and distribution

Several diseases may present with blisters or pustules. There is no common condition that can be used as a "reference point" with which less usual lesions can be compared in the same way as rashes can be compared with psoriasis. A different approach is needed for the assessment of blistering or pustular lesions, based on the history and appearance, and is summarised as the three Ds: development, duration, and distribution.

Development
Was there any preceding systemic illness—as in chickenpox, hand, foot, and mouth disease, and other viral infections? Was there a preceding area of erythema—as in herpes simplex or pemphigoid? Is the appearance of the lesions associated with itching—as in herpes simplex, dermatitis herpetiformis, and eczematous vesicles on the hands and feet?

Duration
Some acute blistering arises rapidly—for example, in allergic reactions, impetigo, erythema multiforme, and pemphigus. Other blisters have a more gradual onset and follow a chronic course—as in dermatitis herpetiformis, pityriasis lichenoides, and the bullae of porphyria cutanea tarda. The rare genetic disorder epidermolysis bullosa is present from, or soon after, birth.

Distribution
The distribution of blistering rashes helps considerably in making a clinical diagnosis. The most common patterns of those that have a fairly constant distribution are shown.

Itching is a very useful symptom. If all the accessible lesions are scratched and it is hard to find an intact blister it is probably an itching rash.

Clinical features: widespread blisters

Chickenpox
Chickenpox is so well known in general practice that it is rarely seen in hospital clinics and is sometimes not recognised. The prodromal illness lasts one to two days and is followed by erythematous lesions that rapidly develop vesicles, then pustules, followed by crusts in two to three days. Crops of lesions develop at the same sites—usually on the trunk, face, scalp, and limbs. The oral mucosa may be affected. The condition is usually benign.

Dermatitis herpetiformis
Dermatitis herpetiformis occurs in early and middle adult life and is characterised by symmetrical, intensely itching vesicles on the trunk and extensor surfaces. The vesicles are superficial. The onset is gradual, but may occur rapidly. The distribution is shown in the diagram.

Variants of dermatitis herpetiformis are larger blisters forming bullae and erythematous papules and vesicles.

Associated conditions
Coeliac disease with villous atrophy and gluten intolerance may occur in association with dermatitis herpetiformis. Linear IgA

The differential diagnosis of blistering eruptions

Widespread blisters
- Eczema—lichenification and crusting, itching
- Dermatitis herpetiformis—itching, extensor surface, persistent
- Chickenpox—crops of blisters, self limiting, prodromal illness
- Pityriasis lichenoides—pink papules, developing blisters
- Erythema multiforme—erythematous and "target" lesions, mucous membranes affected
- Pemphigoid—older patients, trunk, and flexures affected. Preceding erythematous lesions, deeply situated, tense blisters
- Pemphigus—adults, widespread superficial blisters, mucous membranes affected (erosions)
- Drug eruptions—history of drugs prescribed, overdose (barbiturates, tranquillisers)

Localised blisters
- Eczema—"pompholyx" blisters on hand and feet, itching
- Allergic reactions, including topical medication, insect bites
- Psoriasis—deep, sterile, non-itching blisters on palms and soles
- Impetigo—usually localised, staphylococci and streptococci isolated
- Herpes simplex—itching lesions developing turbid blisters

Diseases presenting with blisters and pustules

Itching	Non-itching
Eczema pompholyx on hands and feet	Erythema multiforme
Allergic reactions	Pemphigus vulgaris
Dermatitis herpetiformis	Bullous pemphigoid
Chickenpox	Bullous impetigo
Herpes simplex	Insect bite allergy
	Pustular psoriasis on hands and feet

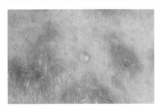

Dermatitis herpetiformis

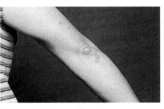

Dermatitis herpetiformis

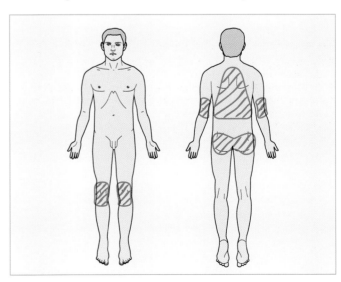

Dermatitis herpetiformis—distribution pattern

disease is a more severe, widespread disease, in which there are "linear" deposits of lgA along the basement membrane of the epidermis and not only at the tips of the papillae as in dermatitis herpetiformis. Treatment is with dapsone or sulfapyridine together with a gluten free diet.

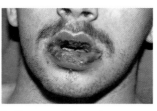

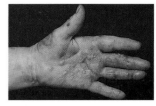

Erythema multiforme in Stevens–Johnson syndrome

Erythema multiforme showing blisters

Erythema multiforme with blisters

Blisters can occur on the lesions of erythema multiforme to a variable degree; when severe, generalised, and affecting the mucous membranes it is known as Stevens–Johnson syndrome. The typical erythematous maculopapular changes develop over one to two days with a large blister (bulla) developing in the centre of the target lesions. In severe progressive cases there is extensive disease of the mouth, eyes, genitalia, and respiratory tract. The blisters are subepidermal, although some basement membrane remains on the floor of the blister.

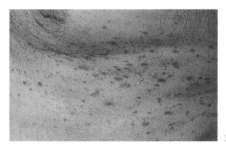

Pityriasis lichenoides

Pityriasis lichenoides varioliformis acuta

As the name implies lichenified papules are the main feature of pityriasis lichenoides varioliformis acuta (or Mucha–Habermann disease), but vesicles occur in the acute form. Crops of pink papules develop centrally, with vesicles, necrosis, and scales—resembling those of chickenpox—hence the "varioliformis". There is considerable variation in the clinical picture, and a prodromal illness may occur. The condition may last from six weeks to six months. No infective agent has been isolated. The pathological changes parallel the clinical appearance with inflammation around the blood vessels and oedema within the dermis.

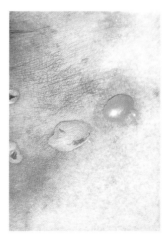

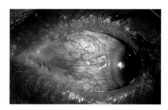

Bullous pemphigoid

Mucous membrane pemphigoid

Pemphigoid

The bullous type of pemphigoid is a disease of the elderly in which tense bullae develop rapidly, often with a preceding erythematous rash, as well as on normal skin. It is mainly seen in the elderly and is slightly more common in women. The flexural aspects of the limbs and trunk and flexures are mainly affected. The bullae are subepidermal and persistent, with antibodies deposited at the dermo-epidermal junction. Unlike pemphigus there is a tendency for the condition to remit after many months.

Another type of pemphigoid occurs in which there is scarring of the oral mucous membrane and the conjunctiva. Occasionally localised lesions are seen on the legs with evidence of an immune reaction, but often the absence of circulating antibasement membrane antibodies. This is a relatively benign condition and often responds to topical steroids.

Treatment is with corticosteroids by mouth, 40–60 mg daily in most patients, although higher doses are required by some. Azathioprine aids remission, with reduced steroid requirements, but takes some weeks to produce an effect. It is essential to check the serum thiopurine methyl transferase (TPMT) level before starting treatment. Patients with low levels have impaired ability to metabolise azathioprine and are likely to suffer toxic effects. Topical steroids can be used on developing lesions.

Chronic scarring pemphigoid affects the mucous membranes with small bullae that break down, leading to erosions and adhesions in the conjunctivae, mouth, pharynx, and genitalia.

There is also a localised type of pemphigoid occurring on the legs of elderly women that runs a benign self-limiting course.

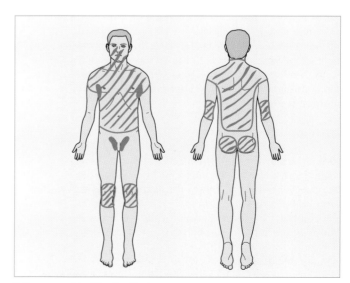

Bullous pemphigoid—distribution pattern

Pemphigus

The most common form of pemphigus vulgaris is a chronic progressive condition with widespread superficial bullae arising in normal skin. In about half of the cases this is preceded by blisters and erosions in the mouth. The bullae are easily broken, and even rubbing apparently normal skin causes the superficial epidermis to slough off (Nikolsky sign). These changes are associated with the deposition of immunoglobulin in the epidermal intercellular spaces. It is a serious condition with high morbidity, despite treatment with steroids and azathioprine. Pemphigus vegetans and pemphigus erythematosus are less common variants.

Differential diagnosis of ulcers in the mouth

- Trauma (dentures)
- Aphthous ulcers
- *Candida albicans* infection
- Herpes simplex
- Erythema multiforme (from drugs)
- Pemphigus
- Lichen planus
- Carcinoma

Clinical features: localised blisters

Pompholyx, which means "a bubble", is characterised by persistent, itchy, clear blisters on the fingers, which may extend to the palms, with larger blisters. The feet may be affected. Secondary infection leads to turbid vesicle fluid. Pompholyx may be associated with a number of conditions—atopy, stress, fungal infection elsewhere, and allergic reactions. It may occur as a result of ingesting nickel in nickel sensitive patients and a similar reaction has been reported to neomycin.

Pustular psoriasis is characterised by deep seated sterile blisters, often with no sign of psoriasis elsewhere—hence the term palmopustular pustulosis. Foci of sepsis have long been considered a causative factor and recent studies have shown a definite association with cigarette smoking. The pattern of HLA antigens indicates that this may be a separate condition from psoriasis.

Bullous impetigo is seen in children and adults. Staphylococci are usually isolated from the blister fluid. The blisters are commonly seen on the face and are more deeply situated than in the non-bullous variety.

Herpes simplex. Primary infection with type 1 virus occurs on the face, lips, and buccal mucosa in children and young adults. Type II viruses cause genital infection. Itching may be severe.

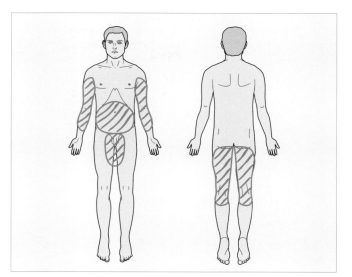

Pemphigus—distribution pattern

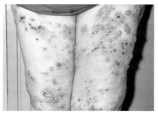

Pemphigus vulgaris

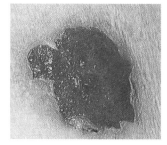

Nikolsky sign

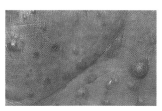

Pompholyx

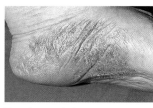

Pustular psoriasis

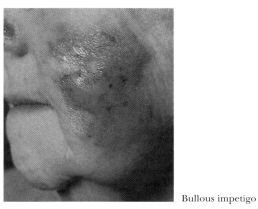

Bullous impetigo

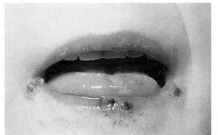

Herpes simplex—type I virus infection

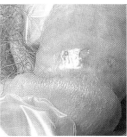

Herpes simplex—type II virus infection

Herpes zoster is due to varicella virus producing groups of vesicles in a dermatome distribution, usually thoracic, trigeminal, or lumbosacral. It is more common after the fourth decade of life.

Insect bite allergy. Large blisters, which are usually not itching, can occur on the legs of susceptible individuals.

Bullous drug eruptions. Fixed drug eruptions can develop bullae, and some drugs can cause a generalised bullous eruption, particularly:

Barbiturates (particularly if taken in overdose)
Sulphonamides
Penicillins
Penicillamine ⎫
Captopril ⎭ pemphigus-like blisters
Frusemide (may be phototoxic)

Remember that there may be an associated erythematous eruption.

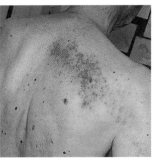
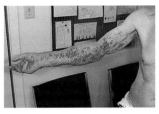

Herpes zoster

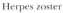

Herpes zoster

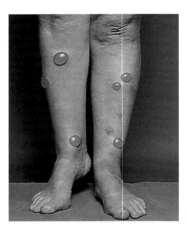

Insect bite allergy

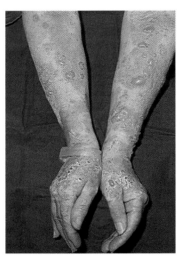

Drug reaction to sulfapyridine

9 Leg ulcers

Although the patient will not probably die of this disease, yet, without great care, it may render her miserable. The disease may be very much relieved by art, and it is one of very common occurrence.

Sir Benjamin Brodie (1846)

Despite the great increase in our understanding of the pathology of leg ulcers, their management is still largely "art". Consequently there are numerous treatments, each with their enthusiastic advocates. There are, however, basic concepts which are helpful in management. As about 95% of leg ulcers are of the "venous" or gravitational variety these will be considered first.

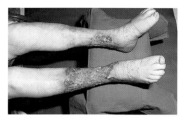
Venous leg ulcers

Pathology of venous ulcers

The skin
Ulcers arise because the skin dies from inadequate provision of nutrients and oxygen. This occurs as a consequence of (a) oedema in the subcutaneous tissues with poor lymphatic and capillary drainage and (b) the extravascular accumulation of fibrinous material that has leaked from the blood vessels. The result is a rigid cuff around the capillaries, preventing diffusion through the wall, and fibrosis of the surrounding tissues.

The blood vessels
Arterial perfusion of the leg is usually normal or increased, but stasis occurs in the venules. The lack of venous drainage is a consequence of incompetent valves between the superficial veins and the deeper large veins on which the calf muscle "pump" acts. In the normal leg there is a superficial low pressure venous system and deep high pressure veins. If the blood flow from superficial to deep veins is reversed then the pressure in the superficial veins may increase to a level that prevents venous drainage, Vancose veins with "back pressure" causing stasis and oedema.

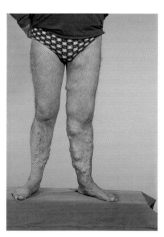
Varicose veins

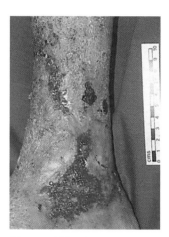
Ulcers and fibrosis

Incompetent valves
Incompetent valves leading to gravitational ulcers may be preceded by:

(1) deep vein thrombosis associated with pregnancy or, less commonly, leg injury, immobilisation, or infarctions in the past
(2) primary long saphenous vein insufficiency
(3) familial venous valve incompetence that presents at an earlier stage—there is a familial predisposition in half of all patients with leg ulcers—or
(4) deep venous obstruction.

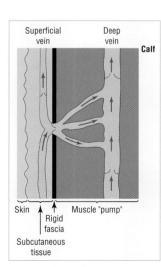
Healthy valves in legs

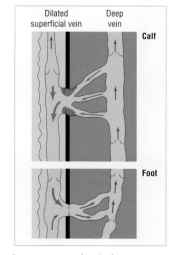
Incompetent valves in legs

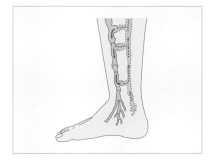
Incompetent flow in legs

43

Who gets ulcers?

Mainly women get ulcers—2% of those over 80 have venous ulcers as a long term consequence of the factors listed above. Leg ulcers are more likely to occur and are more severe in obese people.

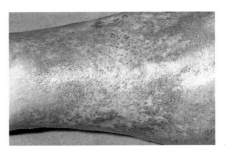

Atrophie blanche

Clinical changes

Oedema and fibrinous exudate often lead to fibrosis of the subcutaneous tissues, which may be associated with localised loss of pigment and dilated capillary loops, an appearance known as "atrophic blanche". This occurs around the ankle with oedema and dilated tortuous superficial veins proximally and can lead to "champagne bottle legs", the bottle, of course, being inverted. Ulceration often occurs for the first time after a trivial injury.

Lymphoedema results from obliteration of the superficial lymphatics, with associated fibrosis. There is often hypertrophy of the overlying epidermis with a "polypoid" appearance, also known as lipodermatosclerosis.

Venous ulcers occur around the ankles, commonly over the medial malleolus. The margin is usually well defined with a shelving edge, and a slough may be present. There may also be surrounding eczematous changes. Venous ulcers are not usually painful but arterial ulcers are.

It is important to check the pulses in the leg and foot as compression bandaging of a leg with impaired blood flow can cause ischaemia and necrosis.

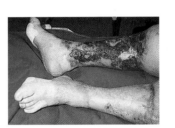

"Champagne bottle legs" with ulceration

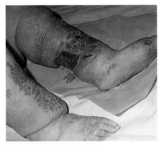

"Champagne bottle legs" with ulceration

Treatment

When new epidermis can grow across an ulcer it will, and the aim is to produce an environment in which this can take place. To this end several measures can be taken:

(1) Oedema may be reduced by means of: (a) diuretics; (b) keeping the legs elevated when sitting; (c) avoiding standing as far as possible; (d) raising the heels slightly from time to time helps venous return by the "calf muscle pump"; (e) applying compression bandages to create a pressure gradient towards the thigh.
(2) Exudate and slough should be removed. Lotions can be used to clean the ulcer and as compresses—0·9% saline solution, sodium hypochlorite solution, Eusol, or 5% hydrogen peroxide.

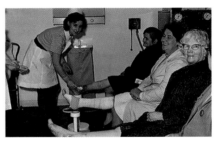

Bandaging

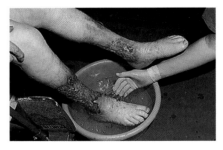

Cleaning the ulcers

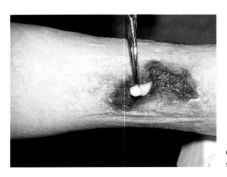

Cleaning with saline solution

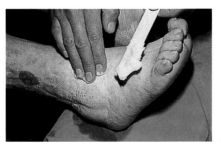

Applying antiseptic cream

There is some evidence that antiseptic solutions and chlorinated solutions (such as sodium hypochlorite and Eusol) delay collagen production and cause inflammation. Enzyme preparations may help by "digesting" the slough. To prevent the formation of granulation tissue use silver nitrate 0·25% compresses, a silver nitrate "stick" for more exuberant tissue, and curettage, if necessary.

(3) The dressings applied to the ulcer can consist of: (a) simple non-stick, paraffin gauze dressings—an allergy may develop to those with an antibiotic; (b) wet compresses with saline or silver nitrate solutions for exudative lesions; (c) silver sulfadiazine (Flamazine) or hydrogen peroxide creams (Hioxyl); and (d) absorbent dressings, consisting of hydrocolloid patches or powder, which are helpful for smaller ulcers.

(4) Paste bandages, impregnated with zinc oxide and antiseptics or ichthammol, help to keep dressings in place and provide protection. They may, however, traumatise the skin, and allergic reactions to their constituents are not uncommon.

(5) Treatment of infection is less often necessary than is commonly supposed. All ulcers are colonised by bacteria to some extent, usually coincidental staphylococci. A purulent exudate is an indication for a broad spectrum antibiotic and a swab for bacteriology. Erythema, oedema, and tenderness around the ulcers suggest a β haemolytic streptococcal infection, which will require long term antibiotic treatment. Dyes can be painted on the edge of the ulcer, where they fix to the bacterial wall as well as the patient's skin. In Scotland bright red eosin is traditionally used, while in the south a blue dye, gentian violet, is favoured. Systemic antibiotics have little effect on ulcers but are indicated if there is surrounding cellulitis. A swab for culture and sensitivity helps to keep track of organisms colonising the area.

(6) Surrounding eczematous changes should be treated. Use topical steroids, not more than medium strength, avoiding the ulcer itself. Ichthammol 1% in 15% zinc oxide and white soft paraffin or Ichthopaste bandages can be used as a protective layer, and topical antibiotics can be used if necessary. It is important to remember that any of the commonly used topical preparations can cause an allergic reaction: neomycin, lanolin, formaldehyde, tars, Chinaform (the "C" of many proprietary steroids).

(7) Skin grafting can be very effective. There must be a healthy viable base for the graft, with an adequate blood supply; natural re-epithelialisation from the edges of the ulcer is a good indication that a graft will be supported. Pinch grafts or partial thickness grafts can be used. Any clinical infection, particularly with pseudomonal organisms, should be treated.

(8) Maintaining general health, with adequate nutrition and weight reduction, is important.

(9) Corrective surgery for associated venous abnormalities.

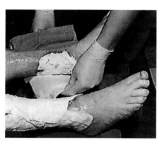

Applying ichthopaste bandages as a protective layer

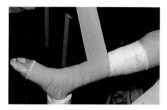

Bandaging ulcers

Treatment of venous leg ulcers

- Take measures to eliminate oedema and reduce weight—make sure the patient understands these
- Never apply steroid preparations to the ulcer itself or it will not heal. Make sure that both nurses and patients are aware of this
- Beware of allergy developing to topical agents—especially to antibiotics
- There is no need to submit the patient to a variety of antibiotics according to the differing bacteria isolated from leg ulcer slough, unless there is definite evidence of infection of adjacent tissue clinically
- A vascular "flare" around the ankle and heel with varicose veins, sclerosis, or oedema indicates a high risk of ulceration developing
- Make sure arterial pulses are present. A Doppler apparatus can be used

Arterial ulcers

Ulcers on the leg also occur as a result of: (a) atherosclerosis with poor peripheral circulation, particularly in older patients; (b) vasculitis affecting the larger subcutaneous arteries; and (c) aterial obstruction in macroglobulinaemia, cryoglobulinaemia, polycythaemia, and "collagen" disease, particularly rheumatoid arthritis.

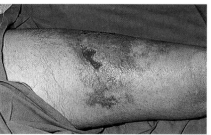

Arterial ulcer

Arterial ulcers are sharply defined and accompanied by pain, which may be very severe, especially at night. The leg, especially the pretibial area, is affected rather than the ankle. In patients with hypertension a very tender ulcer can develop posteriorly (Martorelli's ulcer).

As mentioned above, compression bandaging will make arterial ulcers worse and may lead to ischaemia of the leg.

Diagnosis

The differing presentation of arterial and venous ulcers helps in distinguishing between them, but some degree of aterial insufficiency often complicates venous ulcers.

Phlebography and Doppler ultrasound may help in detecting venous incompetence and arterial obstruction, which can sometimes be treated surgically.

Ulcers on the leg may also occur secondary to other diseases, because of infection, in malignant disease, and after trauma.

Secondary ulcers

Ulcers occur in diabetes, in periarteritis nodosa, and in vasculitis. Pyoderma gangrenosum, a chronic necrotic ulcer with surrounding induration, may occur in association with ulcerative colitis or rheumatoid vasculitis.

Infections

Infections that cause ulcers include staphylococcal or streptococcal infections, tuberculosis (which is rare in the United Kingdom but may be seen in recent immigrants), and anthrax.

Malignant diseases

Squamous cell carcinoma may present as an ulcer or, rarely, develop in a pre-existing ulcer. Basal cell carcinoma and melanoma may develop into ulcers, as may Kaposi's sarcoma.

Trauma

Patients with diabetic or other types of neuropathy are at risk of developing trophic ulcers. Rarely they may be self induced—"dermatitis artefacta".

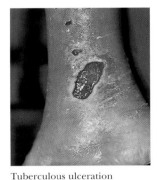

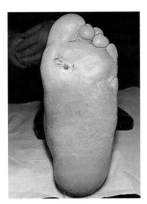

Ulcer in diabetic foot

Tuberculous ulceration

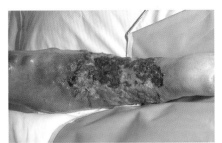

Squamous cell carcinoma in venous ulcer

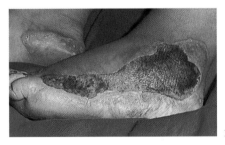

Dermatitis artefacta

Further reading

Browse NL, Burnand KG, Lea M. *Diseases of the veins: pathology, diagnosis and treatment.* London: Edward Arnold, 1988

Kappert A. *Diagnosis of peripheral vascular disease.* Berne: Hauber, 1971

Ryan TJ. *The management of leg ulcers,* 2nd ed. Oxford: Oxford University Press, 1987

10   Acne and rosacea

Acne goes with adolescence, a term derived from the Greek "acme" or prime of life. The young girl who is desperately aware of the smallest comedo and the young man, with his face or back a battlefield of acne cysts and scars, are familiar to us all. Both need treatment and help in coming to terms with their condition.

What is acne?

Acne lesions develop from the sebaceous glands associated with hair follicles—on the face, external auditory meatus, back, chest, and anogenital area. (Sebaceous glands are also found on the eyelids and mucosa, prepuce and cervix, where they are not associated with hair follicles.) The sebaceous gland contains holocrine cells that secrete triglycerides, fatty acids, wax esters, and sterols as "sebum". The main changes in acne are:

(1) an increase in sebum secretion;
(2) thickening of the keratin lining of the sebaceous duct, to produce blackheads or comedones—the colour of blackheads is due to melanin, not dirt;
(3) an increase in *Propionibacterium acnes* bacteria in the duct;
(4) an increase in free fatty acids;
(5) inflammation around the sebaceous gland, probably as a result of the release of bacterial enzymes.

Underlying causes
There are various underlying causes of these changes.

Hormones
Androgenic hormones increase the size of sebaceous glands and the amount of sebum in both male and female adolescents. Oestrogens have the opposite effect in prepubertal boys and eunuchs. In some women with acne there is lowering of the concentration of sex hormone binding globulin and a consequent increase in free testosterone concentrations. There is probably also a variable increase in androgen sensitivity. Oral contraceptives containing more than 50 micrograms ethinyloestradiol can make acne worse and the combined type may lower sex hormone binding globulin concentrations, leading to increased free testosterone. Infantile acne occurs in the first few months of life and may last some years. Apart from rare causes, such as adrenal hyperplasia or virilising tumours, transplacental stimulation of the adrenal gland is thought to result in the release of adrenal androgens—but this does not explain why the lesions persist. It is more common in boys.

Fluid retention
The premenstrual exacerbation of acne is thought to be due to fluid retention leading to increased hydration of and swelling of the duct. Sweating also makes acne worse, possibly by the same mechanism.

Diet
In some patients acne is made worse by chocolate, nuts, and coffee or fizzy drinks.

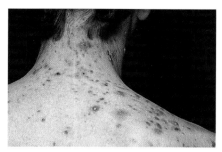
Acne cysts and scars

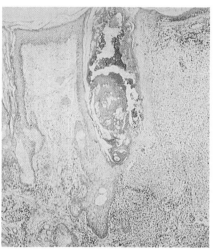
Sebaceous gland—histology of acne

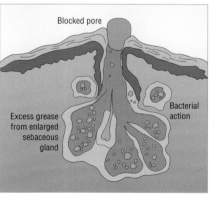
Sebaceous gland—pathology in acne

Hormones—the cause of all the trouble
- Androgens
  - increase the size of sebaceous glands
  - increase sebum secretion
- Androgenic adrenocorticosteroids—have the same effect
- Oestrogens—have the opposite effect

47

Seasons

Acne often improves with natural sunlight and is worse in winter. The effect of artificial ultraviolet light is unpredictable.

External factors

Oils, whether vegetable oils in the case of cooks in hot kitchens or mineral oils in engineering, can cause "oil folliculitis", leading to acne-like lesions. Other acnegenic substances include coal tar, dicophane (DDT), cutting oils, and halogenated hydrocarbons (polychlorinated biphenols and related chemicals). Cosmetic acne is seen in adult women who have used cosmetics containing comedogenic oils over many years.

Iatrogenic factors

Corticosteroids, both topical and systemic, can cause increased keratinisation of the pilosebaceous duct. Androgens, gonadotrophins, and corticotrophin can induce acne in adolescence. Oral contraceptives of the combined type can induce acne, and antiepileptic drugs are reputed to cause acne.

Types of acne
Acne vulgaris • Affects comedogenic areas • Occurs mainly in puberty, in boys more than girls • Familial tendency **Infantile acne** • Face only • Clears spontaneously **Severe acne** • Acne conglobata • Pyoderma faciale • Gram negative folliculitis **Occupational acne** • Oils • Coal and tar • Chlorinated phenols • DDT and weedkillers **Steroids** • Systemic or topical **Hormones** • Combined type of oral contraceptives and androgenic hormones

Types of acne

Acne vulgaris

Acne vulgaris, the common type of acne, occurs during puberty and affects the comedogenic areas of the face, back, and chest. There may be a familial tendency to acne. Acne vulgaris is slightly more common in boys, 30–40% of whom have acne between the ages of 18 and 19. In girls the peak incidence is between 16 and 18 years. Adult acne is a variant affecting 1% of men and 5% of women aged 40. Acne keloidalis is a type of scarring acne seen on the neck in men.

Patients with acne often complain of excessive greasiness of the skin, with "blackheads", "pimples", or "plukes" developing. These may be associated with inflammatory papules and pustules developing into larger cysts and nodules. Resolving lesions leave inflammatory macules and scarring. Scars may be atrophic, sometimes with "ice pick" lesions or keloid formation. Keloids consist of hypertrophic scar tissue and occur predominantly on the neck, upper back, and shoulders and over the sternum.

Acne excoreé

The changes of acne are often minimal but the patient, often a young girl, picks at the skin producing disfiguring erosions. It is often very difficult to help the patient break this habit.

Infantile acne

Localised acne lesions occur on the face in the first few months of life. They clear spontaneously but may last for some years. There is said to be an associated increased tendency to severe adolescent acne.

Acne conglobata

This is a severe form of acne, more common in boys and in tropical climates. It is extensive, affecting the trunk, face, and limbs. In "acne fulminans" there is associated systemic illness with malaise, fever, and joint pains. It appears to be associated with a hypersensitivity to *P. acnes*. Another variant is pyoderma faciale, which produces erythematous and necrotic lesions and occurs mainly in adult women.

Gram negative folliculitis occurs with a proliferation of organisms such as klebsiella, proteus, pseudomonas, and *Escherichia coli*.

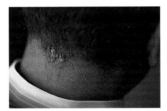
Acne keloidalis

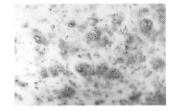
Acne with comedones

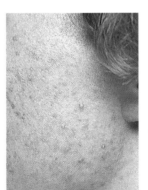
"Ice-pick" scars

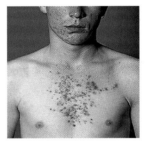
Acne vulgaris

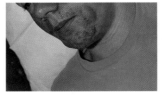
Acne fulminans

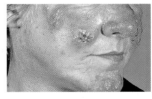
Pyoderma faciale

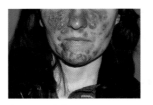
Acne conglobata

Gram negative folliculitis

Occupational

Acne-like lesions occur as a result of long term contact with oils or tar as mentioned above. This usually results from lubricating, cutting, or crude oil soaking through clothing. In chloracne there are prominent comedones on the face and neck. It is caused by exposure to polychlortriphenyl and related compounds and also to weedkiller and dicophane.

Treatment of acne

In most adolescents acne clears spontaneously with minimal scarring. Reassurance and explanation along the following lines helps greatly:

(1) The lesions can be expected to clear in time.
(2) It is not infectious.
(3) The less patients are self conscious and worry about their appearance the less other people will take any notice of their acne.

It helps to give a simple regimen to follow, enabling patients to take some positive steps to clear their skin and also an alternative to picking their spots.

Patients with acne should be advised to hold a hot wet flannel on the face (a much simpler alternative to the commercial "Facial saunas"), followed by gentle rubbing in of a plain soap. Savlon solution, diluted 10 times with water, is an excellent alternative for controlling greasy skin. There are many proprietary preparations, most of which act as keratolytics, dissolving the keratin plug of the comedone. They can also cause considerable dryness and scaling of the skin.

Benzoyl peroxide in concentrations of 1–10% is available as lotions, creams, gels, and washes. Resorcinol, sulphur, and salicylic acid preparations are also available.

Vitamin A acid as a cream or gel is helpful in some patients. A topical tretinoin gel has recently been introduced.

Ultraviolet light therapy is less effective than natural sunlight but is helpful for extensive acne. It is a helpful additional treatment in the winter months.

Oral treatment. The mainstay of treatment is oxytetracycline, which should be given for a week at 1 g daily then 500 mg (250 mg twice daily) on an empty stomach. Minocycline or doxycycline are alternatives that can be taken with food. Perseverance with treatment is important, and it may take some months to produce an appreciable improvement. Erythromycin is an alternative to tetracycline, and co-trimoxazole can be used for Gram negative folliculitis. Tetracycline might theoretically interfere with the absorption of progesterone types of birth control pill and should not be given in pregnancy.

Topical antibiotics. Erythromycin, the tetracyclines, and clindamycin have been used topically. There is the risk of producing colonies of resistant organisms.

Antiandrogens. Cyproterone acetate combined with ethinyloestradiol is effective in some women; it is also a contraceptive.

Synthetic retinoids. For severe cases resistant to other treatments these drugs, which can be prescribed only in hospital, are very effective and clear most cases in a few months. 13-cis-Retinoic acid (isotretinoin) is usually used for acne. They are teratogenic, so there must be no question of pregnancy, and can cause liver changes with raised serum lipid values. Regular blood tests are therefore essential. A three month course of treatment usually gives a long remission. Recently topical isotretinoin gel has been introduced.

Residual lesions, keloid scars, cysts, and persistent nodules can be treated by injection with triamcinolone or freezing with

Treatment of acne

First line	Second line	Third line
Encourage positive attitudes	Topical vitamin A acid	Oral retinoids for 3–4 months (hospitals only)
Avoid environmental and occupational factors	Topical antibiotics	
Topical treatment Benzoyl peroxide Salicylic acid	Ultraviolet light	
A tetracycline by mouth for several months	Antiandrogens	

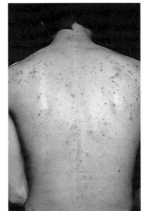
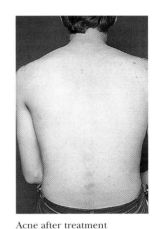

Acne before treatment

Acne after treatment

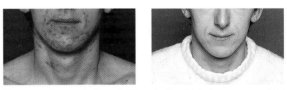

Severe cystic acne before (left) and after (right) treatment with tetracycline

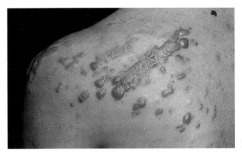

Keloid scars

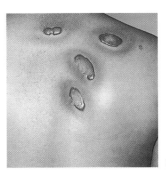

Keloid scars on dark skin

liquid nitrogen. For severe scarring dermabrasion can produce good cosmetic results. This is usually carried out in a plastic surgery unit.

Rosacea

Rosacea is a persistent eruption occurring on the forehead and cheeks. It is more common in women than men.

There is erythema with prominent blood vessels. Pustules, papules, and oedema occur. Rhinophyma, with thickened erythematous skin of the nose and enlarged follicles, is a variant. Conjunctivitis and blepharitis may be associated. It is usually made worse by sunlight.

Rosacea should be distinguished from:

- Acne, in which there are blackheads, a wider distribution, and improvement with sunlight. Acne, however, may coexist with rosacea—hence the older term "acne rosacea".
- Seborrhoeic eczema, in which there are no pustules and eczematous changes are present.
- Lupus erythematosus, which shows light sensitivity, erythema, and scarring but no pustules.
- Perioral dermatitis, which occurs in women with pustules and erythema around the mouth and on the chin. There is usually a premenstrual exacerbation. Treatment is with oral tetracyclines.

Treatment

The treatment of rosacea is with long term courses of oxytetracycline, which may need to be repeated. Topical treatment along the lines of that for acne is also helpful. Topical steroids should not be used as they have minimal effect and cause a severe rebound erythema, which is difficult to clear. Avoiding hot and spicy foods may help.

Recent reports indicate that synthetic retinoids are also effective.

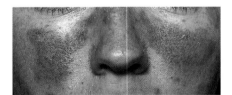

Lupus erythematosus

Remember the following points
- Avoid topical steroids
- Persevere with one antibiotic not short courses of different types
- Do not prescribe a tetracycline for children and pregnant women
- Oxytetracycline must be taken on an empty stomach half an hour before meals

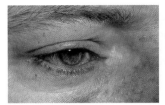

Blepharitis

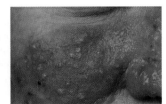

Rosacea

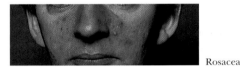

Rosacea

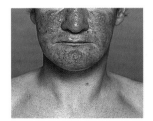

Rosacea

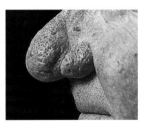

Rhinophyma

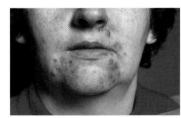

Perioral dermatitis on treatment with cyproterone acetate

Further reading

Cunliffe WJ, Cotterill JA. *The acnes: clinical features, pathogenesis and treatment.* St Louis: Mosby, 1989.
Plewig G, Kligman AM. *Acne and rosacea,* 2nd ed. Berlin: Springer-Verlag, 1992

11 The hair and scalp

D Kemmett

Introduction

Hair, which has an essential physiological role in animals, is mainly of psychological importance in man. A good head of hair provides some degree of warmth for the human head and also protection from ultraviolet radiation, but its significance is otherwise in the eye of the beholder. In the form of wool, hair is of economic importance and considerable research has been carried out into the cycles of growth and the structure of wool keratin in sheep.

Too much hair, particularly on the face of women, is an embarrassment and cosmetic problem and loss of hair from the scalp is equally troublesome. Changes in hair growth are not only of cosmetic significance but can also be associated with underlying diseases. Diseases occurring in the skin of the scalp can damage hair follicles leading to loss of hair. This chapter covers: (a) the normal pattern of hair growth; (b) causes of hair loss; (c) skin diseases involving the scalp; (d) causes of excess hair growth; (e) abnormalities of the hair itself; and (f) treatment.

The normal pattern of hair growth

Unlike other epidermal structures which grow continuously, hair has a cyclical pattern of growth. The growing phase or anagen lasts an average of 1000 days on the scalp followed by an involutional phase known as catagen which is quite short, lasting only a few days. The hair then enters a resting phase, telogen, lasting about 100 days. In man, hair growth is normally asynchronous, with each individual hair following its own cycle independently of the others. The basal layer of the hair bulb from which the hair itself is produced is known as the matrix and contains melanocytes from which melanin pigment is incorporated into the hair. The type of melanin determines the colour and in grey or white hair, pigment production is reduced or absent.

The body surface with the exception of the palms, soles, the lips, and the genitalia, is covered with fine vellus hairs that do not have a medulla and are not pigmented. These hairs develop into longer coarse, medullated, terminal hair on the scalp and eyebrows. At puberty a similar change occurs in the pubic area and the axillae, also on the face and trunk, in the male. These changes are androgen dependent, even in females, but testicular androgen is required to produce beard growth and balding in men.

Racial characteristics and the genetic make-up of the individual determine the type and colour of the hair. Straight black oriental hair is clearly different from the nordic blonde type.

Hair loss

This is known as alopecia, said to be derived from the Latin "alopex", a fox, presumably because of the bald patches of mange seen in wild foxes.

Adult male pattern alopecia is so common as to be considered normal. Circulating levels of testosterone are not

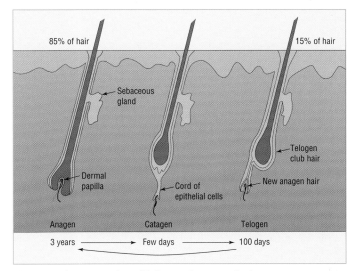

Diagrammatic cross-section of hair at various growth phases

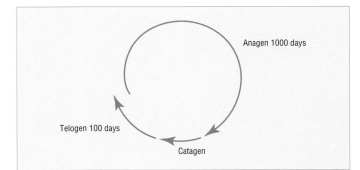

Hair growth cycle

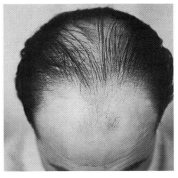

Male pattern baldness

raised in bald men but there is evidence that availability of the hormone to the hair follicle is increased. In postmenopausal women there may be widespread thinning of the hair but loss of hair at the temples often occurs to some degree at an earlier age.

Alopecia may be diffuse or localised. If it is simply due to a physiological derangement of hair growth, the follicles remain intact, whereas inflammation may lead to scarring and loss of the hair follicles. Hence, hair loss can be classified into the categories shown in the illustration on the right.

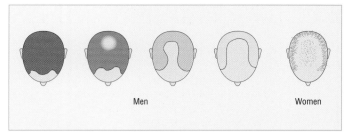

Adult pattern of alopecia: comparison between men and women

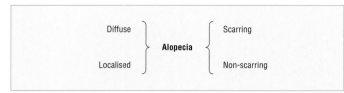

Classification of alopecia

Diffuse hair loss

An interruption of the normal hair cycle leads to generalised hair loss. This may be due to changes in circulating hormones, drugs, inflammatory skin disease, and "stress" of various types.

Telogen effluvium occurs if all the hairs enter into the resting phase together, most commonly after childbirth or severe illness. Two or three months later the new anagen hair displaces the resting telogen hair, resulting in a disconcerting, but temporary, hair loss from the scalp. Stress of any type, such as an acute illness or an operation, causes a similar type of hair loss.

Postfebrile alopecia occurs when a fever exceeds 39 °C, particularly with recurrent episodes. It has been reported in a wide range of infectious diseases, including glandular fever, influenza, malaria, and brucellosis. It also occurs in fever associated with inflammatory bowel disease.

Dietary factors such as iron deficiency and hypoproteinaemia may play a role, but are rarely the sole cause of diffuse alopecia.

Severe malnutrition with a protein deficiency results in dystrophic changes with a reduction in the rate of hair growth.

Congenital alopecia may occur in some hereditary syndromes.

Anagen effluvium occurs when the normal development of hair and follicle is interfered with, resulting in inadequate growth. As a result, hairs are shed earlier than usual, while still in the anagen phase.

Endocrine causes of diffuse alopecia include both hypo- and hyperthyroidism, hypopituitarism, and diabetes mellitus. In hypothyroidism the hair is thinned and brittle, whereas in hypopituitarism the hair is finer and soft but does not grow adequately.

Systemic drugs—cytotoxic agents, anticoagulants, immunosuppressants, and some antithyroid drugs—may cause diffuse hair loss, usually an "anagen effluvium" as mentioned above.

Inflammatory skin disease, when widespread, can be associated with hair loss, for example in erythroderma due to psoriasis or severe eczema.

Deficiency states are a rare cause of alopecia. Patients who suffer from hair loss are often convinced that there is some deficiency in their diet and may sometimes produce the results of an "analysis" of their hairs which show deficiencies in specific trace elements. In fact it is very difficult to cause actual hair loss even in gross malnutrition and in those dying from starvation in refugee camps, the hair growth in the scalp is usually

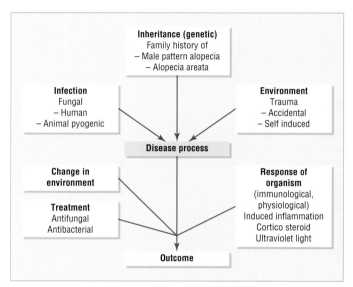

Factors leading to development of alopecia

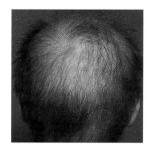

Anagen effluvium

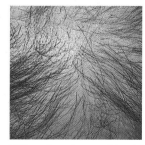

Diffuse alopecia caused by ciclosporin

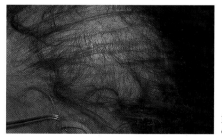

Diffuse alopecia caused by erythrodermic psoriasis

present. In chronic malnutrition or kwashiorkor, the hair assumes a curious red/brown colour which may be due to iron deficiency.

Treatment

Wherever possible, the cause should be treated. This may be a matter of replacement therapy in hormonal deficiency. In alopecia due to stress, once this cause is removed hair growth may revert to normal. Treatment of inflammatory skin disease will result in some improvement of the hair loss.

Androgenic alopecia in men is best accepted, with assurance that it indicates normal virility.

Minoxidil causes hair growth and is commercially available as a lotion. This has to be applied continuously every day as the scalp reverts to a level of loss which would have occurred without treatment as soon as it is stopped. It is effective in about half the patients with male pattern alopecia.

Localised alopecia

Alopecia areata is a common form of hair loss. It is seen in 2% of patients attending the average dermatology clinic in the United Kingdom. There may be small patches of hair loss or the whole scalp may be affected. Resolution occurs in a few months or the condition may persist for years. There may be slight inflammation of the skin in the affected areas—in keeping with the possibility of an underlying immune reaction against the hair follicles. There is also an association with autoimmue disease and atopy.

In the affected areas the follicles are visible and empty. The hairs about to be lost have an "exclamation mark" appearance and in some areas that are resolving, fine vellus hairs are seen. Patches commonly occur on the scalp, face, or eyebrows. In *alopecia totalis*, the whole head is involved, and in *alopecia universalis* hair is lost from the whole of the body.

In many patients, particularly if it is a first episode, regrowth occurs within a few months with fine pale hairs appearing first, being replaced by normal adult hair. In older patients, non-pigmented hair may persist in previous patches of alopecia. Factors associated with a poor prognosis are:

(1) Repeated episodes of alopecia
(2) Very extensive or complete hair loss (alopecia totalis)
(3) Early onset before puberty
(4) In association with atopy

Differential diagnosis includes trauma from the habit of plucking hair (trichotillomania) in mentally disturbed patients and traction alopecia from tight hair rollers or hair styles that involve tension on the hair. In fungal infections (tinea capitis) there is scaling and broken hairs. Fungal spores or hyphae are visible in hair specimens on microscopy.

Inflammation is present with loss of hair follicles in lupus erythematosus and lichen planus.

Treatment

An initial limited area of alopecia areata in adult life can be expected to regrow and treatment is generally not needed. Treatments that are carried out include:

(1) Injection of triamcinolone diluted with local anaesthetic which usually stimulates localised regrowth of hair. Unfortunately it often falls out again and there is a risk of causing atrophy. Topical steroid lotion can be used but results are variable.

Causes of diffuse non-scarring alopecia

Androgenetic alopecia
- Male pattern
- Female pattern

Endocrine-thyroid disease (hypothyroidism and hyperthyroidism)
- Hypopituitarism
- Diabetes mellitus

Stress
- Postpartum
- Postoperative   } telogen effluvium
- Postfebrile

Drugs
- Cytotoxics
- Anticoagulants
- Antithyroid agents   } anagen effluvium
- Ciclosporin

Erythrodermic skin disease
- Psoriasis
- Eczema
- Inflammatory

Deficiency states
- Protein malnutrition
- Iron deficiency

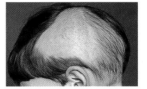

Alopecia areata

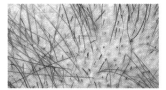

Alopecia areata, showing exclamation mark hairs

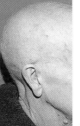

Alopecia totalis

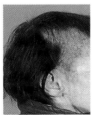

Trichotillomania

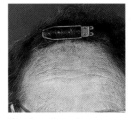

Traction alopecia

(2) Ultraviolet light or psoralen with ultraviolet A can give good, if transient, results in a few patients but it has little effect in the majority. It may act by suppressing an immune reaction around the hair root.

(3) Induced contact dermatitis and irritants are occasionally effective. Cantharadin and dithranol have been used for many years as irritants. Primula leaves or chemicals (for example, diphencyprone) can be applied to produce an acute contact dermatitis. The mechanism by which acute inflammation stimulates hair growth is not understood.

Scarring alopecia

The absence of hair follicles is an important physical sign as it indicates:

(1) The presence of an inflammatory process that requires further investigation.
(2) That there is unlikely to be any substantial recovery of hair growth.

The presence of inflammation does not necessarily produce marked erythema—in lichen planus and lupus erythematosus, the inflammatory changes are often chronic. Systemic lupus erythematosus produces areas of inflammation that extend, leaving residual scarring. In discoid lupus erythematosus there is more scaling with keratotic plugs in the follicle. Localised scleroderma (morphoea) also causes alopecia, often with a linear atrophic lesion—the *en coup de sabre* pattern.

More acute inflammatory changes are seen as a result of pyogenic infection or kerion in which there is a marked inflammatory reaction to fungal infection from cattle. In "folliculitis decalvans" there is florid folliculitis with deep seated pustules and scarring. Treatment is with prolonged antibiotics.

Tinea capitis can be associated with alopecia.

Trauma can also cause scarring with alopecia.

Skin disease involving the scalp

The scalp can be involved in any skin disease, but most commonly in psoriasis and seborrhoeic eczema. A mild degree of scaling from accumulation in skin scales is so common as to be normal (dandruff). Increased accumulation of scales is seen in seborrhoeic dermatitis in which pityrosporum organisms may play a part. Sometimes masses of thick adherent scales develop in *pityriasis amiantacea*, usually due to psoriasis. Eczema and contact dermatitis can also involve the scalp.

Aetiological factors in alopecia areata

Genetic
- Familial in about 20% of cases
- Associated with Down's syndrome

Immunological
- T lymphocytic infiltrate around hair follicles
- Associated with autoimmune disease

Stress
- May be associated in individual patients

Causes of scarring alopecia

Trauma
- For example, burns

Inflammation
Acute
- bacterial (pyogenic infection, syphilis)
- viral (herpes simplex, herpes zoster, varicella)
- fungal (keroin caused by animal ringworm)

Chronic
- lupus erythematosus
- lichen planus
- folliculitis decalvans
- morphoea

Rare
- pyoderma gangrenosum
- necrobiosis lipoidica
- sarcoidosis

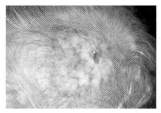
Scarring in lupus erythematosus

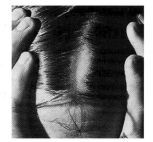
En coup de sabre pattern in alopecia

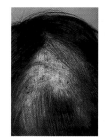
Folliculitis decalvans

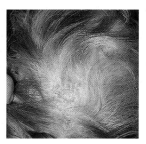
Tinea capitis

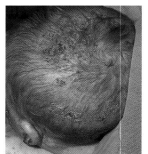
Atopic eczema

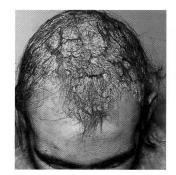
Pityriasis amiantacea

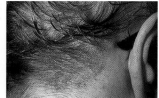
Contact eczema, hair dye

Treatment

Scaling and inflammatory changes can be improved with the use of sulphur and salicylic ointment. It is effective but messy and best applied at night. Tar preparations, oil of cade, and coconut oil in various formulations are all effective. Topical steroids can also be used to suppress inflammation.

Hair shaft abnormalities

Congenital abnormalities of the hair shaft itself lead to weak, thin and broken hairs. In some cases there is a characteristic appearance, for example "spun glass" appearance of pili torti with a twisted hair. In monilethrix there are regular nodes in the hair shaft.

There are other abnormalities of the hair shaft which are not associated with increased fragility, such as the Willi hair syndrome, progressive kinking of the hair and uncombable hair, in which the hair grows in disorderly profusion, completely resistant to combing and brushing. In pili annulati there may be a spangled appearance due to bright bands in the hair shaft.

Excessive hair

Two types of overgrowth of hair occur:

Hirsuties

This is the growth of coarse terminal hair in a male distribution occurring in a woman. This is not always easy to assess since what is unacceptable and emotionally disturbing to one woman may be quite acceptable to another. The amount of hair growth may appear to be within normal limits in a patient complaining of excessive hair but it should never be dismissed as of no consequence if it is important to the woman concerned. Nevertheless, it is important to limit the number of investigations once it is clear that there is no underlying abnormality. Strong reassurance may then be the most helpful management. It is of course most apparent on the face but is often present on the thighs, abdomen and back as well.

Hirsuties occurs most commonly after the menopause and may be present to some degree in normal women as a result of familial or racial traits. It may arise without any underlying hormonal disorder or as a result of virilising hormones. These causes are listed in the box on the right. In addition to androgens, a number of drugs can cause hirsuties. It is important to remember that hirsuties may be part of a virilising syndrome or polycystic ovaries. It is useful to measure the serum testosterone and oestrogen level, as well as urinary 17 oxosteroid concentrations.

Hypertrichosis

This is an excessive growth of hair which may be generalised or localised. It may be due to metabolic disturbance or drugs, or simply a feature of a localised lesion such as a mole.

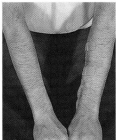

Hypertrichosis caused by minoxidil

Cutaneous diseases of the scalp

Common

Inflammatory
- Psoriasis
- Seborrhoeic eczema
- Contact dermatitis

Infection
- Folliculitis—staphylococcal or streptococcal
- Fungal infection
    Microsporum, with hair loss
    Trichophyton, with scaling and inflammation
- Herpes—zoster and simplex

Infestation
- Pediculosis

Less common
- Lupus erythematosus
- Lichen planus
- Pemphigoid and pemphigus

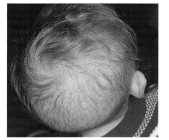

Monilethrix

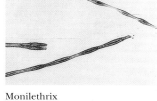

Monilethrix

Causes of hirsutism

Hereditary, racial with wide variation of normal pattern

Endocrine

Adrenal
- Virilising tumours
- Cushing's syndrome
- Adrenal hyperplasia

Ovarian
- Virilising tumours
- Polycystic ovary syndrome

Pituitary
- Acromegaly
- Hyperprolactinaemia

Iatrogenic
- Anabolic steroids
- Androgens, corticosteroids
- Danazol, phenytoin
- Psoralens (in psoralen with ultraviolet A)

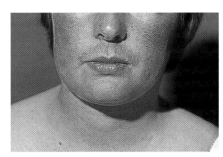

Hirsuties due to virilising tumour

Treatment

It is clearly important to treat any underlying cause and this will usually improve the condition. Otherwise treatment is symptomatic and includes:

- Removal of hair by shaving or hair removing creams.
- Electrolysis and diathermy, which gives permanent destruction of the hair follicle.
- Antiandrogen drugs such as cyproterone can be used under specialist supervision.

Causes of hypertrichosis

- Naevoid—in pigmented naevi and Becker's naevus
- Congenital (rare)
- Acquired—porphyria, hyperthyroidism, anorexia nervosa some developmental defects, for example, Hurler's syndrome, tumours (hypertrichosis lanuginosa), drugs (diazoxide, minoxidil, ciclosporin)

Further reading

Orfanos CE, Happle R. *Hair and hair disease.* Berlin: Springer-Verlag, 1990

Rook A, Dawber R. *Diseases of the hair and scalp,* 3rd ed. Oxford: Blackwell Scientific, 1997

12 Diseases of the nails

AL Wright

In animals and birds claws are used for digging and grasping as well as for fighting. The human nail may be used as a weapon but its main function is to protect the distal soft tissues of the fingers and toes.

As an ectodermal derivative composed of keratin, the nail plate grows forward from a fold of epidermis over the nail bed which is continuous with the matrix proximally. The keratin composing the nail is derived mainly from the matrix with contributions from the dorsal surface of the nail fold, and the nail bed also adds keratin to the deep surface.

The nail grows slowly for the first day after birth then more rapidly until it slows in old age. The rate of nail growth is greater in the fingers than the toes, particularly on the dominant hand. It is slower in women but increases during pregnancy. Finger nails grow at approximately 0·8 mm per week and toe nails 0·25 mm per week.

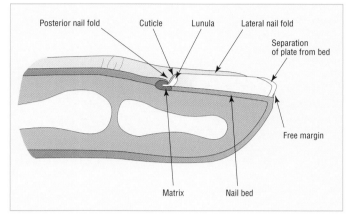

Section through finger showing nail structure

Physical signs in the nails

The changes in the nail may be due to a local disease process, a manifestation of a skin disease, or a systemic disorder. Hereditary disorders may also affect the nails. It is therefore important to take both a general history and specifically enquire about skin diseases. It sometimes happens that the nail changes are the only sign of a dermatological disease, although the patient may have a previous history of lichen planus or psoriasis, for example. Localised infection or trauma will affect one or two nails. Skin disease, such as psoriasis, affects many or all nails, usually symmetrically, whereas systemic illness or drugs will affect all the nails.

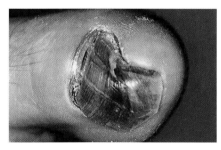

Effect of trauma

Local nail changes

Trauma
- Acute trauma. This may remove the whole nail.
- Chronic trauma as a result of badly fitting footwear may cause thickening of the nail with deformed growth, onychogryphosis. Chronic trauma due to overenthusiastic manicuring or habitual picking at finger nails can result in deformity and impaired growth.
- Repeated trauma in occupations that involve repetitive action, such as assembling cardboard boxes, may cause detachment of the nail (*onycholysis*) or splitting of the nails.

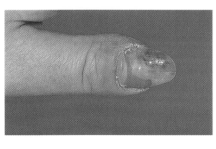

Paronychia

Infection
- Infection of the tissues around the nail (*paronychia*) is often mixed with pyogenic organisms, including pseudomonas, as well as yeasts such as candida. This condition occurs most frequently in those employed in the food industry and occupations where there is repeated exposure to a moist environment and minor trauma. The index and middle fingers are most frequently involved.
- Infection of the nail plate itself occurs in fungal infections, which are commonly due to *Trichophyton* or *Epidermophyton* species.

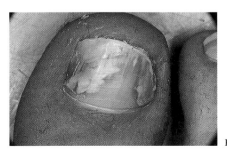

Fungal infection

- Those living in the tropics may acquire infection with *Scopulariopsis brevicaulis*, which produces a black discoloration of the nail.

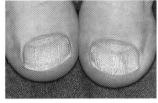
Pitting of nail

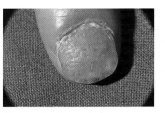
Lichen planus

Skin diseases affecting the nails

Since the nail plate consists of specialised keratin produced by basal cells, it is not surprising that it is affected by skin diseases. Some conditions, such as psoriasis, may produce characteristic changes whereas in other conditions, such as eczema, the changes are much less specific.

Psoriasis causes an accumulation of keratin, as in lesions of the skin. This may result in the nail being both thickened and raised from the nail bed (*onycholysis*). There may be the changes of pustular psoriasis in the surrounding tissues, indistinguishable from acrodermatitis pustulosa. Loss of minute plugs of abnormal keratin results in "pitting".

Lichen planus produces atrophy of the nail plate which may completely disappear. The cuticle may be thickened and grow over the nail plate, known as *pterygium formation*.

Eczema may be associated with brittle nails that tend to split. Thickening and deformity of the nail occurs in eczema or contact dermatitis, sometimes with horizontal ridging.

Darier's disease results in dystrophy of the nail and longitudinal streaks which end in triangular-shaped nicks at the free edge. On the skin there may be the characteristic brownish scaling papules on the central part of the back, chest, and neck. These are made worse by sun exposure.

Alopecia areata is quite often associated with changes in the nails including ridges, leuconychia, and friable nails. It may be associated with "20 nail dystrophy".

Autoimmune conditions such as pemphigus and pemphigoid may be associated with a variety of changes including ridging, splitting of the nail plate, and atrophy in some or all of the nails.

Discoloration of the nail and friability are associated with *lupus erythematosus*.

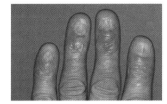
Dystrophy due to lupus erythematosus

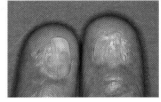
Pterygium formation due to lichen planus

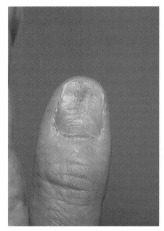
Nail dystrophy

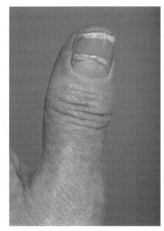
Beau's line

General diseases affecting the nails

Nail changes in systemic illness
Acute illness results in a transverse line of atrophy known as a Beau's line. Shedding of the nail, *onychomedesis*, may occur in severe illness.

Chronic diseases
Clubbing affects the soft tissues of the terminal phalanx with swelling and an increase in the angle between the nail plate and the nail fold. It is associated with chronic respiratory disease, cyanotic heart disease, and occasionally in chronic gastrointestinal conditions. It is occasionally hereditary and may be unilateral in association with vascular abnormalities.

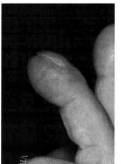
Clubbing

Colour changes
All the nails may be *white* (leukonychia) due to hypoalbuminaemia in conditions such as cirrhosis of the liver. Brown discoloration is seen in renal failure and the "*yellow nail syndrome*", may be associated with abnormalities of the lymphatic drainage. The nail may have a yellow colour in jaundice. *Drugs* may cause changes in colour, for example tetracycline may produce yellow nails, antimalarials a blue

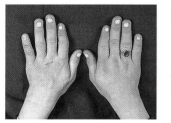
Leukonychia

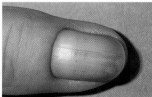
Yellow nail syndrome

discolouration, and chlorpromazine a brown colour. Leuconychia or whiteness of the nails occurs in fungal infections. Small white spots on the nail are quite commonly seen and are thought to be due to trauma of the nail plate.

Longitudinal pigmented streaks result from increased melanin deposition in the nail plate.

Longitudinal brown streaks are frequently seen in individuals with racially pigmented skin, particularly after trauma. This is rare in caucasians but occurs as a result of a benign pigmented naevus at the base of the nail and in associated lentigo. The most important cause to remember is *subungual melanoma*, which may present with a longitudinal deep brown or black streak. Hutchinson's sign with pigmentation extends into the surrounding tissues, particularly the cuticle. Adrenal disease may rarely be associated with longitudinal streaks.

Specific changes in the nail plate

Thickening
This may be due to:

- Hyperkeratosis—psoriasis; fungal infection
- Hypertrophy—chronic trauma (onychogryphosis); pachyonychia congenita
- Atrophy lupus erythematosus—lichen planus; congenital dystrophy.

Thickening of the nail plate may be due to hyperkeratosis in psoriasis, in which case the changes will be symmetrical and there may well also be pitting of the nail and onycholysis. Similar changes are seen in fungal infection of the nail, which may be symmetrical on the toes. Nail clippings should be sent for microscopy and mycological culture.

Hypertrophy of the nail plate occurs as a result of chronic trauma, with only a few nails affected, and is usually seen in the feet.

Pachyonychia congenita is a rare congenital disorder characterised by hypertrophic nails.

Hyperkeratosis, due to the accumulation of keratin under the nail plate, is also seen in psoriasis. It occurs occasionally in association with chronic dermatitis.

Detachment of the nail plate (onycholysis)
- Psoriasis
- Fungal infection
- Trauma
- Thyrotoxicosis.

Onycholysis is due to a detachment of the nail from the nail bed. If it is extensive, there may be complete loss of the nail plate. It is most commonly seen in psoriasis and occasionally in fungal infections of the nail. It may occur as a result of trauma or thyrotoxicosis

Pitting of the surface of the nail plate
- Psoriasis
- Alopecia

Pitting of the nail plate is due to punctate depressions on the surface of the nail plate. They are most often seen in psoriasis but may occur in alopecia areata.

Horizontal ridging
- Beau's lines may be seen after systemic illness and acute episodes of hand dermatitis.

Pigmented streaks

Malignant melanoma
Normal in pigmented skin
- Melanocytic naevi
- Lentigo
- Addison's disease

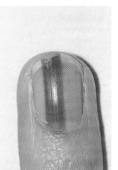
Melanocystic naevus

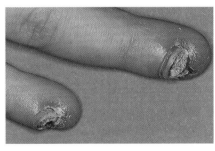
Psoriasis

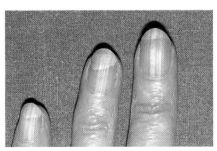
Onycholysis due to psoriasis

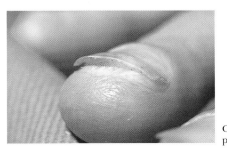
Onycholysis due to psoriasis

Longitudinal ridging
- Single due to pressure from nail fold tumours
- Multiple due to lichen planus
- Alopecia areata
- Psoriasis
- Darier's disease.

Ridging represents a disturbance of nail growth. Inflammation as seen in acute paronychia or trauma can result in a single nail developing a horizontal ridge. After an acute illness there may be horizontal lines on all the nails. The lines may also occur with eczema.

A single longitudinal ridge can result from pressure due to benign or malignant tumours in the nail fold. A mucoid cyst can produce a longitudinal ridge. Multiple longitudinal lines are characteristic of lichen planus, psoriasis, alopecia areata, and Darier's disease.

Koilonychia is a concave deformity of the nail plate, generally occurring in the finger nails. It may be idiopathic or occur as a result of iron deficiency anaemia.

Lesions adjacent to the nail

Mucoid cysts develop subcutaneously over the distal interphalangeal joint and may be adjacent to the nail, producing abnormalities of growth. These cysts develop as an extension of the synovial membrane and are linked to the joint by a fine tract. Very careful excision is required for a cure.

Naevi may occur adjacent to the nail and a benign melanocytic naevus can produce a pigmented streak. Subungual melanoma may produce considerable pigmentation of the nail and often causes pigmentation of the cuticle, so called Hutchinson's sign. Sometimes subungual melanoma is amelanotic so there is no pigmentary changes and any rapidly growing soft tumour should raise suspicions of this condition.

Subungual exostosis can cause a painful lesion under the nail. It is confirmed by x ray examinations.

Glomus tumours arise as tender nodules.

Periungual fibrokeratomas also develop in patients with tuberous sclerosis.

Treatment of nail conditions

It is clearly not possible to treat congenital abnormalities of the nail, but avoiding exposure to trauma may help. Nail changes associated with dermatological conditions may improve as the skin elsewhere is treated. Systemic treatment of associated dermatoses will of course tend to improve the nail as well, for example methotrexate or retinoids for psoriasis.

Infective lesions respond to antifungal or antibiotic treatment. In chronic paronychia there is often a mixed infection and a systemic antibiotic combined with topical nystatin may be required. It is also important to keep the hands as dry as possible.

The imidazole antifungal drugs are fairly effective but are fungistatic. Terbinaline is fungicidal and a short course is as effective as prolonged treatment with the older drug griseofulvin.

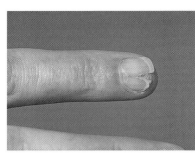
Darier's disease

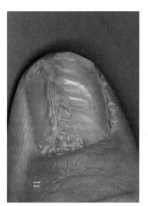
Longitudinal ridge

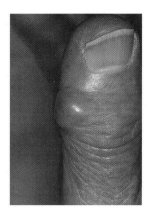
Mucoid cyst

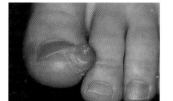

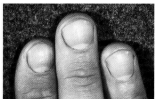
Big toe exostosis

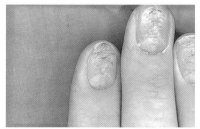
Nail dystrophy with alopecia areata

Nail dystrophy with eczema

Further reading

Baden HP. *Diseases of the hair and nails.* Chicago: Year Book Medical, 1986

Baran R. *Nail disorders: common presenting signs, differential diagnosis and treatment.* Edinburgh: Churchill Livingstone, 1991

De Berker DA, Baran R, Dawber RP. *Handbook of diseases of the nails and their management.* Oxford: Blackwell Scientific, 1995

13   Lumps and bumps

The skin is a common site for neoplastic lesions, but most invade only locally and with treatment usually do not pose any threat to the life of the patient. The exception is malignant melanoma, which is dealt with in chapter 15. This is a rare tumour with a high mortality, and recent publicity campaigns have been aimed at preventing the tragedy of fatal metastases from a neglected melanoma.

As a result a large number of patients are being seen with pigmented skin lesions and nodules, only a very few of which are neoplastic. The question is how to distinguish the benign, the malignant, and the possibly malignant. The following guidelines may help in deciding whether the lesion can be safely left or should be treated.

A correlation of the clinical and pathological features is helpful in making a confident diagnosis of the more common tumours.

Seborrhoeic warts

Seborrhoeic warts come in various shapes, sizes, and colours. When deeply pigmented, inflamed, or growing they may appear to have the features of a malignant lesion, but the following features are characteristic:

- Well defined edge.
- Warty, papillary surface—often with keratin plugs.
- Raised above surrounding skin to give a "stuck on" appearance.

Individual lesions vary considerably in size, but are usually 0·5–3·0 cm in diameter. Protuberant and pedunculated lesions occur. Solitary lesions are commonly seen on the face and neck but more numerous, large lesions tend to occur on the trunk. They become more common with increasing age.

Basal cell carcinoma

By contrast, the early basal cell carcinoma—or rodent ulcer—presents as a firm nodule, clearly growing within the skin and below it, rather than on the surface. The colour varies from that of normal skin to dark brown or black, but there is commonly a "pearly" translucent quality. As its name implies, the tumour is composed of masses of dividing basal cells that have lost the capacity to differentiate any further. As a result no epidermis is formed over the tumour and the surface breaks down to form an ulcer, the residual edges of the nodule forming the characteristic "rolled edge". Once the basal cells have invaded the deeper tissues the rolled edge disappears.

Variants

Variants of the usual pattern can cause problems in diagnosis. Cystic basal cell carcinomas occur, and those that show differentiation towards hair follicles or sweat glands may

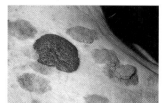

Seborrhoeic wart

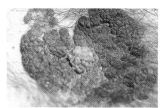

Seborrhoeic wart

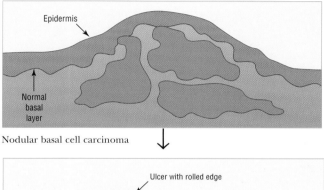

Nodular basal cell carcinoma

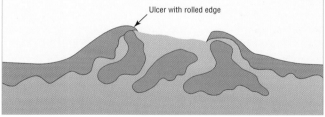

Ulcerated basal cell carcinoma

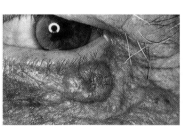

Clumps of neoplastic basal cells

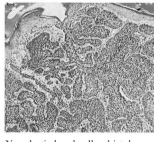

Neoplastic basal cells—histology

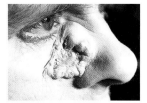

Basal cell carcinoma (later stage of figure above)

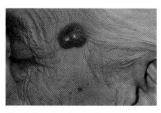

Cystic basal cell carcinoma

have a less typical appearance. Pigmented lesions can resemble melanoma. The superficial spreading type may be confused with a patch of eczema. This usually occurs on the trunk, does not itch, and shows a gradual but inexorable increase in size. A firm "whipcord" edge may be present. The sclerosing type has scarring of the epidermis associated with basal cell carcinoma.

Treatment

Various methods of destroying tumour tissue are used and the results are similar for radiotherapy and surgical excision:

- Ulcerated lesions may invade tissue planes, blood vessels, and nerves more extensively than is clinically apparent.
- Although modern techniques of radiotherapy result in minimal scarring and atrophy these may cause problems near the eye.
- Basal cell carcinomas in skin creases, such as the nasolabial fold, tend to ulcerate and are hard to excise adequately.
- Surgical excision has the advantage that should the lesion recur, radiotherapy is available to treat it, whereas it is not desirable to treat recurrences after radiotherapy with further irradiation.

Squamous cell carcinoma

Squamous cell carcinoma represents proliferation of the epidermal keratinocytes in a deranged manner—with a visible degree of differentiation into epidermal cells that may show individual cell keratinisation and "pearls" of keratin. In other tumours bizarre cells with mitoses, cells with clear cytoplasm, or spindle cells may be seen.

This type of cancer often develops from a preceding solar keratosis or an area of Bowen's disease. They may also complicate a chronic ulcer due to stasis, as in venous ulcer of the ankle, or infection such as leprosy or tuberculosis. In addition to local spread, metastases can occur with involvement of other organs such as the liver, lung or brain, and lymphadenopathy. The first change clinically is a thickening of the skin with scaling or hyperkeratosis of the surfaces. The more differentiated tumours often have a warty, keratotic crust whereas others may be nodular. The edge is poorly defined. There may be associated dilated, telangiectatic blood vessels. The original hard, disc-like lesion becomes nodular and ulcerates with strands of tumour cells invading the deeper tissue. The thick warty crust, often found elsewhere, may be absent from the lesions on the lip, buccal mucosa, and penis.

These histological changes complement the clinical appearance and are clearly different from those of basal cell carcinoma.

Treatment

Small lesions should be excised as a rule, making sure that the palpable edge of the tumour is included, with a 3–5 mm margin. Radiotherapy is effective but fragile scars may be a disadvantage on the hand. Cryotherapy or topical fluorouracil can be used for histologically confirmed, superficial lesions and also for solar keratoses.

Solar keratoses

Solar keratoses occur on sites exposed to the sun and are more common in those who have worked out of doors or sunbathed excessively. The common sites are the face, back of the hands,

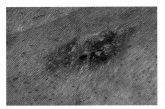
Superficial basal cell carcinoma

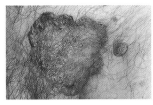
Pigmented basal cell carcinoma

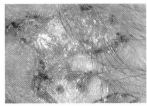
Sclerosing basal cell carcinoma

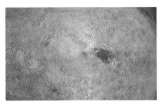
Squamous cell carcinoma—initial changes

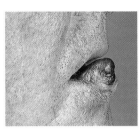
Squamous cell carcinoma—more differentiated tumour

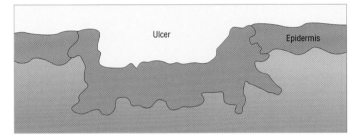
Squamous neoplastic cells

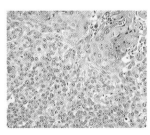
Squamous cell carcinoma—histological appearance

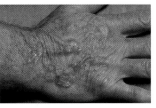
Solar keratoses

arms, and legs. They also develop on the scalp in bald men and on the lips, particularly in pipe smokers. They show alterations in keratinisation and have the potential to become dysplastic and eventually develop into squamous cell carcinoma, a change often preceded by inflammation. They can be regarded as squamous cell carcinoma grade 1/2.

The clinical appearance varies from a rough area of skin to a raised keratotic lesion. The edge is irregular and they are usually less than 1 cm in diameter. Inflammation and tenderness may be associated with progression to carcinoma.

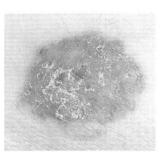

Bowen's disease

Treatment

Treatment with cryotherapy, using liquid nitrogen or carbon dioxide, repeated if necessary, is usually effective.

5-Fluorouracil cream is useful for larger or multiple lesions. It is applied twice daily for two weeks, which produces inflammation and necrosis. Simple dressings are applied for the next two weeks. This process can be repeated if necessary. As it is a cytotoxic drug it should be handled with care and applied sparingly with a cotton bud while wearing gloves.

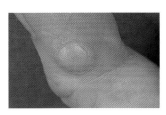

Paget's disease of the nipple

Other conditions

Bowen's disease is characterised by a well defined, erythematous macule with little induration and slight crusting. It is a condition of the middle aged and elderly, occurring commonly on the trunk and limbs. It is an intraepidermal carcinoma, which has been reported to follow the ingestion of arsenic in "tonics" taken in years gone by or exposure to sheep dip, weedkiller, or industrial processes. After many years florid carcinoma may develop with invasion of deeper tissues. It may be confused with a patch of eczema or superficial basal cell carcinoma. Lesions on covered areas may be associated with underlying malignancy. Erythroplasia of Queyrat is a similar process occurring on the glans penis or prepuce.

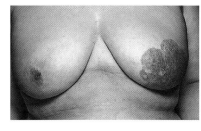

Keratoacanthoma

Paget's disease of the nipple presents with unilateral non-specific erythematous changes on the aureola and nipple, spreading to the surrounding skin. The cause is an underlying adenocarcinoma of the ducts. It should be considered in any patient with eczematous changes of one breast that fail to respond to simple treatment. Extramammary lesions occur.

Keratoacanthoma is a rapidly growing fleshy nodule that develops a hard keratotic centre. Healing occurs with some scarring. Although benign, it may recur after being removed with curette and cautery, particularly from the face, and is best excised.

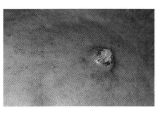

Dermatofibroma

Benign tumours

Dermatofibroma is a simple, discrete firm nodule, arising in the dermis at the site of an insect bite or other trivial injury. Often there is a brown or red vascular lesion initially, which then becomes fibrotic—a sclerosing haemangioma. The histiocytoma is similar but composed of histiocytes.

Skin tags may be pigmented but rarely cause any diagnostic problems unless inflamed. Some are in fact pedunculated seborrhoeic warts and others simple papillomas (fibroepithelial polyps).

Lipomas are slow growing benign subcutaneous tumours.

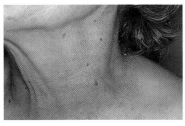 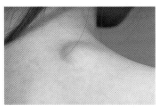

Skin tags   Lipoma

Other benign tumours

A wide variety of tumours may develop from the hair follicle and sebaceous, exocrine (sweat), and apocrine glands. The more common include *syringomas*—slowly growing, small, multiple nodules on the face of eccrine gland origin.

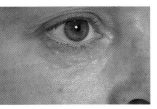

Syringoma

Naevus sebaceous is warty, well defined, varying in size from a small nodule to one several centimetres in diameter. Lesions occur in the scalp of children, may be present at birth, and gradually increase in size. They may proliferate or develop into a basal cell carcinoma in adult life and they are therefore best removed.

Verrucous epidermal naevi are probably a variant, found on the trunk and limbs.

Cysts

The familiar *epidermoid cyst*—also known as sebaceous cyst or wen—occurs as a soft, well defined, mobile swelling usually on the face, neck, shoulder, or chest. It is not derived from sebaceous glands but contains keratin produced by the lining wall.

Pilar cysts on the scalp are similar lesions derived from hair follicles.

Milia are small keratin cysts consisting of small white papules found on the cheek and eyelids.

Vascular lesions

The more common vascular naevi are described.

The *port wine stain*, or naevus flammeus, presents at birth as a flat red lesion, usually on the face, neck, or upper trunk. There is usually a sharp midline border on the more common unilateral lesions. In time the affected area becomes raised and thickened because of proliferation of vascular and connective tissue. If the area supplied by the ophthalmic or maxillary divisions of the trigeminal nerve is affected there may be associated angiomas of the underlying meninges with epilepsy—Sturge–Weber syndrome. Lesions of the limb may be associated with arteriovenous fistulae.

Cavernous angioma—strawberry naevi—appear in the first few weeks of life or at birth. A soft vascular swelling is found, most commonly on the head and neck. The lesions resolve spontaneously in time and do not require treatment unless interfering with visual function.

Spider naevus consist of a central vascular papule with fine lines radiating from it. They are more common in children and women. Large numbers in a man raise the possibility of liver disease.

Campbell de Morgan spots are discrete red papules 1–5 mm in diameter. They are more common on the trunk.

Pyogenic granuloma is a lesion that contains no pus but is in fact vascular and grows rapidly. It may arise at the site of trauma. Distinction from amelanotic melanoma is important.

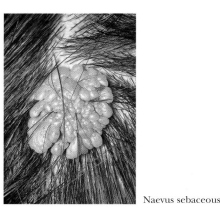
Naevus sebaceous

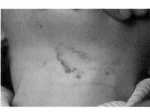
Verrucous epidermal naevus

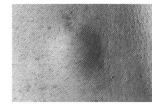
Epidermoid cyst

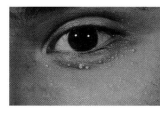
Milia

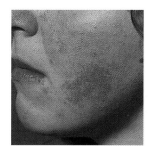
Naevus flammeus

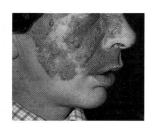
Sturge–Weber syndrome

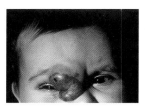
Cavernous angioma in a five month old baby

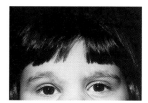
Patient five years later without treatment

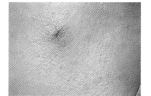
Spider naevi

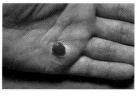
Pyogenic granuloma

Further reading

Enzinger F, Weiss S. *Soft tissue tumours*, 2nd ed. St Louis: Mosby, 1988

Mackie RM. *Skin cancer: an illustrated guide to the etiology, clinical features, pathology and management of benign and malignant cutaneous tumours*, 2nd ed. London: Martin Dunitz, 1996

14 The sun and the skin

R StC Barnetson

People with darkly pigmented skin very rarely get skin cancer. Those of a Celtic constitution, when exposed to strong sunlight in countries such as Australia, get skin cancer very readily. Australia has the highest incidence of skin cancer in the world, with 140 000 new cases per year, and 1200 deaths per year, mainly from melanoma.

It is therefore important to understand that there is a variation in skin sensitivity to sunlight. This is rated from one to six (Fitzpatrick classification). Skin type one subjects have red hair and do not tan, burn very easily in the sun and develop skin cancer readily, whereas skin type six subjects have black skin (with an inbuilt sun protection factor of 10) and very rarely develop skin cancer. This is a useful guide in assessing the risk of sun damage and in determining the dose of ultraviolet B in treatment.

Ultraviolet radiation

There are three types of ultraviolet radiation—the short wavelength ultraviolet C (100–280 nm), ultraviolet B (290–320 nm), and long wavelength ultraviolet A (320–400 nm). Beyond this is visible light then infrared, and radiowaves. ultraviolet C does not penetrate beyond the stratosphere as it is absorbed by the ozone layer. Ultraviolet B is very important in both sunburn and the development of skin cancer. Ultraviolet A is thought to be of increasing importance in the development of skin cancer, and causes tanning but not sunburn. It is also important in people with photosensitivity. The effects of ultraviolet radiation may be classified as short term (sunburn, photosensitivity) or long term (skin cancer, wrinkling, solar elastosis, solar keratoses, seborrhoeic warts).

There is general awareness that the sun causes cancer in the skin, with some people becoming obsessively fearful of any exposure to sun. A sensible approach with emphasis on reasonable precautions is called for. Useful points are:

- Most moles are entirely harmless.
- Detecting the changes in moles or early melanoma enables the diagnosis to be made at an early stage with a good chance of curative treatment.
- The non-melanotic, epidermal cancers—basal cell and squamous cell carcinomas—grow slowly and are generally not life threatening. But squamous cell carinoma arising at sites of trauma, on the extremities, or in ulcers may metastasise. Exposure to sun has usually occurred many years previously.

Prevention of sun damage and skin cancer

Prevention of sun damage and skin cancer will depend on reducing exposure to ultraviolet radiation. This can be achieved in a number of ways:

- Covering the skin with clothes. It must be remembered however that light clothes such as shirts or blouses may only have a sun protection factor of four. A wide-brimmed hat is essential to protect the face and neck.
- Sunscreens will greatly reduce sun exposure for exposed parts such as the face and hands. Sunscreens are much more

Skin types and sun
- Type 1—Never tans, freckles, red hair, blue eyes
- Type 2—Tans with difficulty, less freckled
- Type 3—Tans easily, dark hair, brown eyes
- Type 4—Always tans, Mediterranean skin
- Type 5—Brown skin (for example, Indian)
- Type 6—Black skin (for example, African)

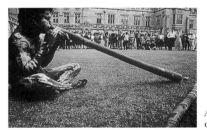
Aborigines do not get skin cancer

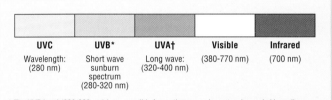

UVC	UVB*	UVA†	Visible	Infrared
Wavelength: (280 nm)	Short wave sunburn spectrum (280-320 nm)	Long wave: (320-400 nm)	(380-770 nm)	(700 nm)

* The UVB band (280-320 nm) is responsible for erythema, sunburn, tanning and skin malignancy
† UVA light (320-400 nm) has the greatest penetration into the dermis and augments UVB erythema and perhaps skin malignancy

Light spectrum (UVC=ultraviolet C, UVB=ultraviolet B, UVA=ultraviolet A)

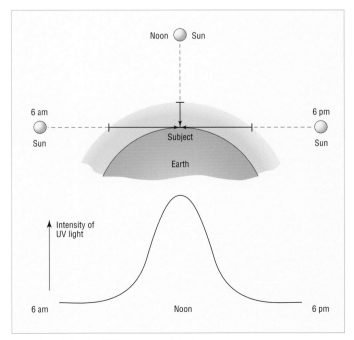
Diurnal variation in UV intensity of light from sun

efficient than previously, particularly those with a sun protection factor greater than 30; they are now water resistant, and most have a broad spectrum, protecting against ultraviolet B and ultraviolet A. This is important because there is now increasing evidence that ultraviolet A is important in the development of skin cancer.

- Exposure to midday sun, particularly in tropical or subtropical latitudes, should be avoided. At this time of the day the sunlight passes vertically through the atmosphere and there is less filtering of dangerous ultraviolet light. So remember the adage: "Between eleven and three, stay under a tree" in the summer months.

Effects of sun
Short term
• Sunburn
• Photosensitivity
Long term
• Skin wrinkling
• Telangiectasia
• Hyper and hypopigmentation
• Solar elastosis
• Actinic keratosis
• Seborrhoeic warts
• Skin cancers

Development of skin cancers

Sun-damaged skin
A number of different features characterise sun-damaged skin, which is often seen in the elderly particularly if they have lived in a sunny climate such as Australia. The skin has many fine wrinkles and often has a sallow yellowish discoloration particularly on the face and other exposed parts of the body. Hyperpigmentation occurs as result of recent sun exposure, which may be diffuse or localised in the form of solar lentigo. In some areas there may be hypopigmentation, particularly where solar keratoses have been treated with liquid nitrogen (cryotherapy). There may be marked telangiectasia and numerous blood vessels are seen. In some, there may be thickening and a yellow hue of the skin, particularly of the neck, due to elastin deposition in the upper dermis; this is known as solar elastosis.

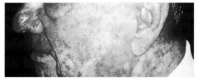
Sun damaged skin

Forms of skin cancer
There are three common forms of skin cancer caused by ultraviolet light: basal cell carcinoma, squamous cell carcinoma, and malignant melanoma. Whereas there seems to be a direct relationship with the amount of ultraviolet exposure and basal cell carcinoma and squamous cell carcinoma, the relationship with ultraviolet exposure and melanoma is more complex and it seems likely that intermittent exposure to ultraviolet light is the main factor (for example, exposure to sunlight on holidays). These different types of neoplastic change that occur in the skin are discussed in chapters 13 and 15.

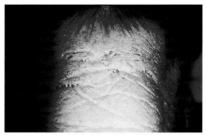
Solar elastosis

Photosensitivity

Exposure to sun in non-pigmented races causes inflammation in the skin, depending on the skin type and amount of exposure. In some individuals there is an abnormal sensitivity to sunlight. This may arise because of an idiopathic reaction to sunlight or allergic reaction that is activated by sunlight. Some chemicals seen to induce photosensitivity without causing an allergy. Other causes are metabolic diseases and inflammatory conditions that are made worse by sun exposure.

Causes of photosensitivity
• Idiopathic—for example, polymorphic light eruption, actinic prurigo, solar urticaria
• Photoaggravated dermatoses—for example, lupus erythematosus, eczema
• Metabolic—porphyria—for example, erythropoietic, hepatic
• Drug induced—for example, sulphonamides, phenothiazines
• Chemical induced (topical)—for example, tar, anthracene

Polymorphic light eruption
This is the most common of the idiopathic photosensitive rashes and occurs predominantly in women. It is due to both the shorter (ultraviolet B) and longer (ultraviolet A) wavelength types of sunlight. The eruption occurs from hours to days after exposure and varies in severity from a few inflamed papules to extensive inflamed oedematous lesions. There may be only a few trivial lesions initially, but increasingly severe reactions can develop restricting the patients ability to venture outside. A useful measure of seventy is to ask the

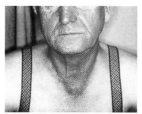
Photosensitivity caused by drugs

patient if they cross to the shady side of the street to avoid the sun. Treatment includes topical or systemic steroids for the acute rash and prevention by using sunscreens. Desensitisation by narrow waveband phototherapy before exposure is effective.

Solar urticaria

This is a much less common condition and may be induced by longer wavelength (ultraviolet A) and visible radiation as well as ultraviolet B. It is characterised by rapidly developing irritation and in the exposed skin is followed by urticarial wheals. It can occur as part of a photoallergic reaction, in which case avoidance of the relevant allergen will prevent the condition.

Treatment is with antihistamines and sunscreens. In some cases phototherapy with ultraviolet B, narrow waveband or psoralen with ultraviolet A (PUVA), is helpful.

15   Black spots in the skin

There has been a great increase in public awareness of melanoma, and any dark lesions of the skin are sometimes regarded with the same dread as Long John Silver's "black spot" in *Treasure Island*—a sign of imminent demise. However, the vast majority of pigmented lesions are simply moles or harmless pigmented naevi. The most important thing is to know which moles can be safely ignored and which should be removed. Benign moles are described first, then malignant melanoma, followed by a discussion of the differences between these two.

Benign moles

Benign moles are naevi with a proliferation of melanocytes and a variable number of dermal naevus cells. Some moles are congenital and are present from birth, but most develop in early childhood and adolescence. The number of moles remains constant during adult life with a gradual decrease from the sixth decade onwards.

There is often an increase in both the number of moles and the degree of pigmentation during pregnancy.

Acquired melanocytic naevi

Acquired melanocytic naevi are the familiar moles and present in a number of different ways depending on the type of cells and the depth in the skin.

Junctional naevi are flat macules with melanocytes proliferating along the dermo-epidermal border.

Compound naevi have pigmented naevus cells at the dermo-epidermal border and in the dermis, producing a raised brown lesion. The dermal melanocytes may accumulate around the skin appendages and blood vessels and form a band of cells without melanin or more deeply penetrating strands of spindle cells. Proliferating naevus cells may throw the overlying epidermis into folds, giving a papillary appearance.

In a purely *intradermal naevus* the junctional element is lost, with the deeper cells showing characteristics of neural tissue. Other types of acquired pigmented naevi include the following.

Blue naevus is a collection of deeply pigmented melanocytes situated deep in the dermis, which accounts for the deep slate-blue colour.

Spitz naevus presents as a fleshy pink papule in children. It is composed of large spindle cells and epitheloid cells with occasional giant cells, arranged in "nests". It is benign and the old name of juvenile melanoma should be abandoned.

Halo naevus consists of a melanocytic naevus with a surrounding halo of depigmentation associated with the presence of antibodies against melanocytes in some cases. The whole naevus gradually fades in time.

Becker's naevus is an area of increased pigmentation, often associated with increased hair growth, which is usually seen on the upper trunk or shoulders. It is benign.

Freckles or ephelides are small pigmented macules, less than 0·5 cm in diameter, that occur in areas exposed to the sun in fair skinned people. These macules fade during the winter months.

Congenital pigmented naevi

Congenital pigmented naevi are present at birth, generally over 1 cm in diameter, and vary from pale brown to black in colour. They often become hairy and more protuberant, possibly with

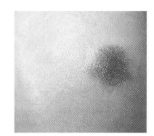
Benign mole

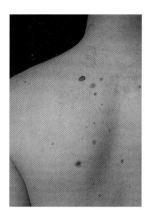
Benign moles

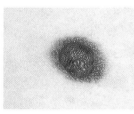
Benign pigmented naevus

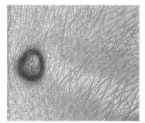
Blue naevus

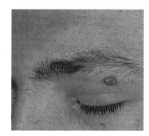
Spitz naevus

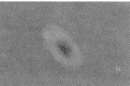
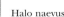
Halo naevus

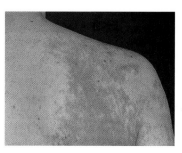
Becker's naevus

an increased risk of malignant change. Larger lesions can cover a considerable area of the trunk and buttocks, such as the bathing trunk naevi, and their removal may present a considerable problem.

Dysplastic naevi

These show very early malignant change and may progress to malignant melanoma. They are deeply pigmented often with an irregular margin.

In *dysplastic naevus syndrome* multiple pigmented naevi that occur predominantly on the trunk, becoming numerous during adolescence. They vary in size—many being over 0·5 cm—and tend to develop into malignant melanoma, particularly if there is a family history of this condition.

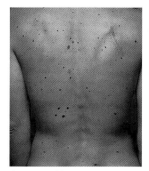

Congenital hairy naevus

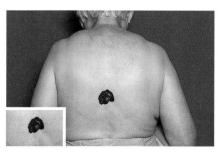

Dysplastic naevus syndrome

Melanoma

Melanoma is an invasive malignant tumour of melanocytes. Most cases occur in white adults over the age of 30, with a predominance in women.

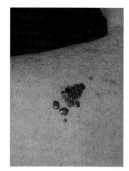

Melanoma

Incidence

The incidence of melanoma has doubled over the past 10 years in Australia (currently 40/100 000 population) and shown a similar increase in other countries. In Europe twice as many women as men develop melanoma—about 12/100 000 women and 6/100 000 men.

Prognosis

The prognosis is related to the thickness of the lesion, measured histologically in millimetres from the granular layer to the deepest level of invasion. Lesions less than 0·76 mm thick have a 100% survival at five years, 0·76–1·5 mm thick an 80% survival at five years, and lesions over 3·5 mm less than 40% survival. These figures are based on patients in whom the original lesion had been completely excised. A recent study in Scotland has shown an overall five year survival of 71·6–77·6% for women and 58·7% for men.

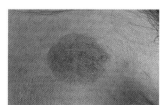

Benign lentigo

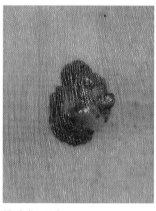

Nodular melanoma

Sun exposure

The highest incidence of melanoma occurs in countries with the most sunshine throughout the year. However, skin type and the regularity of exposure to sun are also important. The incidence is much greater in fair skinned people from higher latitudes who have concentrated exposure to sun during holidays than in those with darker complexions who have more regular exposure throughout the year. Severe sunburn may also predispose to melanoma.

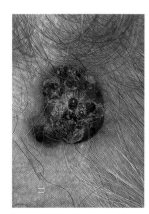

Superficial melanoma with nodules

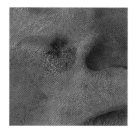

Lentigo maligna

Genetic factors

Since melanin protects the skin from ultraviolet light it is not surprising that melanoma occurs most commonly in fair skinned people who show little tanning on exposure to sun, particularly those of Celtic origin. Members of families with the dysplastic naevus syndrome are more likely to develop melanoma in their moles. These patients have multiple naevi from a young age.

Pre-existing moles

It is rare for ordinary moles to become malignant but congenital naevi and multiple dysplastic naevi are more likely to develop into malignant melanoma.

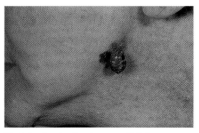

Nodule developing in superficial spreading melanoma

Types of melanoma

There are four main types of melanoma.

Superficial spreading melanoma is the more common variety. It is common on the back in men and on the legs in women. As the name implies the melanoma cells spread superficially in the epidermis, becoming invasive after months or years. The margin and the surface are irregular, with pigmentation varying from brown to black. There may be surrounding inflammation and there is often clearing of the central portion. The invasive phase is associated with the appearance of nodules and increased pigmentation. The prognosis is correspondingly poor.

Lentigo maligna melanoma occurs characteristically in areas exposed to sun in elderly people. Initially there is a slowly growing, irregular pigmented macule that is present for many years before a melanoma develops.

Nodular melanoma presents as a dark nodule from the start without a preceding in situ epidermal phase. It is more common in men than women and is usually seen in people in their fifties and sixties. Because it is a vertical invasive growth phase from the beginning there is a poor prognosis.

Acral melanoma occurs on the palm and soles and near or under the nails. Benign pigmented naevi may also occur in these sites and it is important to recognise early dysplastic change by using the criteria set out below. A very important indication that discoloration of the nail is due to melanoma is Hutchinson's sign—pigmentation of the nail fold adjacent to the nail. It is important to distinguish talon noir, in which a black area appears on the sole or heel. It is the result of trauma—for example sustained while playing squash—causing haemorrhage into the dermal papillae. Paring the skin gently with a scalpel will reveal distinct blood filled papillae, to the relief of doctor and patient alike.

Other types of melanoma

As the melanoma cells become more dysplastic and less well differentiated they lose the capacity to produce melanin and form an amelanonitic melanoma. Such non-pigmented nodules may be regarded as harmless but are in fact extremely dangerous.

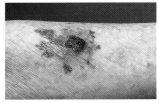

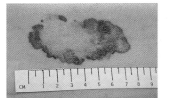

Superficial spreading melanoma

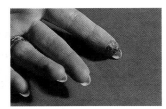

Nodular melanoma in a lentigo

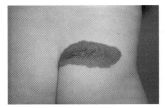

Benign lentigo

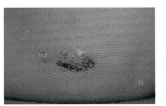

Acral melanoma

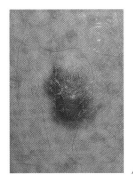

Talon noir of left heel

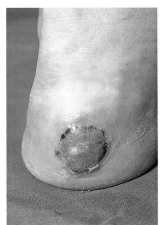

Dysplastic melanoma

Amelanotic melanoma

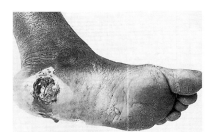

Malignant melanoma in a black person; note the surrounding "halo"

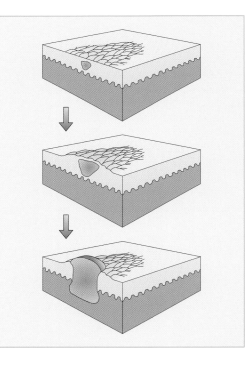

Progressive growth in depth of malignant melanoma

Prognosis

This depends on the depth to which the melanoma has penetrated below the base of the epidermis—lesions confined to the epidermis having better prognosis than those penetrating into the dermis. The Clark classification describes the depth of penetration as follows:

Level I—within the epidermis
Level II—few melanoma cells within the dermal papillae
Level III—many melanoma cells in the papillary dermis
Level IV—invasion of the reticular dermis
Level V—invasion of the subcutaneous tissues

The Breslow classification is based on measurements of tumour thickness from the granular layer overlying epidermis. A depth of less than 1·5 mm is associated with a 90% five year survival, 1·5–3·5 mm with a 75% five year survival, and greater than 3·5 mm with only a 50% five year survival.

In deeper tumours "sentinel lymph node" biopsy may be carried out to assess whether lymphatic spread has occurred.

How to tell the difference

Benign moles show little change and remain static for years. Any change may indicate that a mole is in fact a melanoma or that a mole is becoming active. Size, shape, and colour are the main features and it is change in them that is most important. Patients with moles should have these changes explained to them, in particular that they indicate activity of the cells, not necessarily malignant change.

Criteria for suspecting malignant changes in pigmented lesions

- Growth—Benign pigmented naevi continue to appear in adolescents and young adults. Any mole increasing in size in an adult over the age of 30 may be a melanoma
- Shape—Moles usually have a symmetrical, even outline, any indentations being quite regular; melanomas usually have an irregular edge with one part advancing more than the others
- Colour—Variation in colour of benign moles is even but a melanoma may be intensely black or show irregular coloration varying from white to slate blue, with all shades of black and brown. Inflammation may give a red colour as well. The amelanotic melanoma shows little or no pigmentation
- Size—Apart from congenital pigmentation naevi most benign moles are less than 1 cm in diameter. Any lesion growing to over 0·5 cm should be carefully checked
- Itching—Normally a mole does not itch but a melanoma may. Irritated seborrhoeic warts also itch
- Bleeding and *crusting* occur in an actively growing melanoma

If more than two of these features are present refer the patient for specialist opinion

A simple summary:

A—Asymmetry of the lesion   C—Variations in colour
B—Irregularity of the border   D—Diameter larger
                                       than 0·5 cm

Further reading

Ackerman AB. *Malignant melanoma and other melanocytic neoplasms.* Baltimore: Williams and Wilkins, 1984
Mackie R (ed). *Primary and secondary prevention of malignant melanoma.* Basle: Karger
Roses DF. *Diagnosis and management of cutaneous malignant melanoma.* Philadelphia: Saunders, 1983
Seigler HE. *Clinical management of melanoma.* The Hague: Nijhoff, 1982

16   The skin and systemic disease—Genetics and skin disease (JA Savin)

When a man has on the skin of his body a swelling or an eruption or a spot... and the disease appears to be deeper than the skin it is a leprous disease.

Leviticus 13: 2–3

In ancient times changes in the skin were taken to indicate that the whole body was diseased and although arguments continue about what the Old Testament writers understood by "leprous", there was clearly an appreciation of the connection between the skin and systemic illness. Clinical signs in the skin may give valuable diagnostic clues to underlying disease. The cutaneous signs of systemic disease is a very large subject; and what follows is only an outline of the more common skin changes that may be associated with systemic illness.

A disease affecting internal organs may produce the same changes in both the skin and other organs—as in the connective tissue diseases. However, underlying conditions may be associated with skin changes brought about by quite different processes, as in acanthosis nigricans or dermatomyositis in which there is an underlying neoplasm with characteristic skin signs. Sometimes severe skin disease itself may be the cause of generalised illness.

The skin is also a common site for allergic reactions to drugs, with a rash being the first clinical sign. The florid skin lesions of AIDS illustrate the results of infections when the immune response is impaired.

Conditions affecting both the skin and the internal organs

Immune reactions

Allergic reactions to drugs such as penicillin can occur. In this case the penicillin molecule attaches to serum protein. This compound acts as an antigen and may form a complex with IgG antibody. It is this complex which attaches to blood vessel walls to produce an inflammatory reaction. This presents as a rash developing a few days to two weeks after treatment on the skin, but if it occurs in the kidneys the resulting tissue damage can have serious consequences. This is an example of Type III allergy with antigen–antibody complexes being deposited in the small blood vessels. Sometimes a much more acute anaphylactic reaction develops A fixed drug eruption is characterised by a localised patch of erythema that flares up whenever the drug is taken. Erythema multiforme can occur in drug reactions.

Connective tissue diseases involve complex immunological processes that affect both internal organs and the skin. This means that it is particularly important to realise the significance of any associated skin changes.

Lupus erythematosus

This condition has been described as "a disease with a thousand faces" because of the wide range of organs involved

When to suspect an underlying systemic disease

- An unusual rash which does not have the features of one of the common primary inflammatory skin conditions
- Evidence of systemic illness—weight loss, and other symptoms such as breathlessness, altered bowel function or painful joints
- Erythema of the skin due to inflammation around the blood vessels, usually without epidermal changes—reactive erythema. Vasculitis, in which there are palpable erythematous lesions which may be painful or nodular
- Unusual changes in pigmentation or texture of the skin
- Palpable dermal lesions that may be due to granuloma, metastases, lymphoma, or deposits of fat or minerals

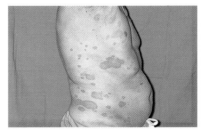
Rash from penicillin

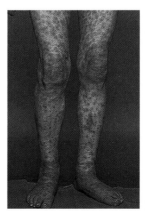
Erythema multiforme

and the numerous ways in which it can present. In three quarters of the patients the skin is involved. There are four main types, with numerous variations.

In *systemic lupus erythematosus* (SLE) the commonest skin change is an acute erythematous eruption occurring bilaterally on the malar area of the face in a "butterfly" distribution. There may also be photosensitivity, hair loss, and areas of vasculitis in the skin. There is often intolerance of sunlight. It is more common in females with a female:male ratio of 8:1.

The systemic changes include fever, arthritis and renal involvement, but there may be involvement of a wide range of organs. The criteria for diagnosing the condition include at least four of the features in the box on the right.

Subacute lupus erythematosus is a variant in about 10% of patients with lupus erythematosus that presents with non-scarring erythematosus plaques mainly on the face, hands and arms. Papulo squamous lesions also occur. They may be annular. Systemic involvement is less common and severe than in SLE. It is associated with a high incidence of neonatal lupus erythematosus in children born to mothers with the condition. The antinuclear factor test is positive in 60% and anticytoplasmic antibodies are present in 80% of patients.

Discoid lupus erythematosus (DLE) is a condition in which circulating antinuclear antibodies are very rare. There are quite well defined photosensitive inflammatory lesions, with some degree of atrophy and hyperkeratosis of the follicles, giving a "nutmeg grater" feel. It occurs predominantly on the face or areas exposed to the sun, becoming worse in the summer months. Scarring is common causing hair loss in lesions on the scalp.

Treatment of SLE with the threatened or actual involvement of other organs is important. Prednisolone is usually required and sometimes immunosuppressant drugs such as azathioprine as well. Treatment of DLE is generally with topical steroids. Hydroxychloroquine by mouth is also used, generally in a dose of 200 mg daily. This drug can diminish visual acuity in higher doses and this should be checked every few months. A simple chart, the Amsler Chart, is available for patients to use, consisting of a central dot with a grid which becomes blurred when held at arm's length when there is any impairment of acuity.

Dermatomyositis

This condition is associated in adults with underlying carcinoma—commonly of the breasts, lung, ovary, or gastrointestinal tract. It is characterised by localised erythema with a purple hue (heliotrope), predominantly on the eyelids, cheeks, and forehead. There may be similar changes on the dorsal surface of the fingers, often with dilated nail fold capillaries. These changes may precede the discovery of an underlying tumour and may also fade away once it is removed. There is a variable association with muscle discomfort and weakness, mainly in the upper limb girdle. The finding of muscle weakness together with specific electromyographic changes and an inflammatory infiltrate in the muscle means there is almost certainly an underlying malignancy, so suitable investigation is indicated.

Systemic sclerosis

As the name implies, there is extensive sclerosis of the connective tissue of the lungs, gastrointestinal tract, kidneys, and heart. Endothelial cell damage in the capillaries results in fibrosis and sclerosis of the organs concerned. The skin becomes tethered to the subcutaneous tissues and immobile, leading to fixed claw like hands, constricted mouth with furrowed lips, and beak-like nose. There are vascular changes producing Raynaud's phenomenon and telangiectasia around

Clinical variants of lupus erythematosus
- Systemic
- Subacute cutaneous
- Discoid (neonatal)
- Systemic sclerosis

Criteria for diagnosing systemic lupus erythematosus
- Malar rash
- Discoid plaques
- Photosensitivity
- Arthritis
- Mouth ulcers
- Renal changes
- Serositis
- Neurological involvement
- Haematological changes
- Immunological changes
- Antinuclear antibodies

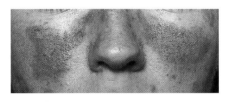
Systemic lupus erythematosus

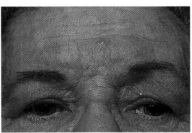
Dermatomyositis

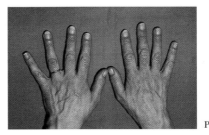
Persistent dermatomyositis

the mouth and on the fingers. There are also flat "mat-like" telangiectasia on the face.

Workers manufacturing polyvinyl chloride can develop skin changes similar to systemic sclerosis with erosions of the bones, hepatic and pulmonary lesions. Pesticides and epoxy resin can also produce scleroderma-like changes.

It is associated with antinuclear antibodies (speckled or nucleolar), and in about 50% of cases, circulating immune complexes may be present.

A variant is the *CREST syndrome*. In this type of scleroderma there is **C**alcinosis with calcium deposits below the skin on the fingers and toes, **R**aynaud's phenomenon with poor peripheral circulation, immobility of the o**E**sophagus, dermal **S**clerosis of the fingers and toes, and **T**elangiectasia of the face and lips and adjacent to the toe and finger nails. It has a better prognosis than systemic sclerosis. Antinuclear antibodies at the centromere are frequently present.

Morphoea is a benign form of localised systemic sclerosis in which there is localised sclerosis with very slight inflammation. There is atrophy of the overlying epidermis. The early changes often consist of a dusky appearance to the skin.

Lichen sclerosus

The full name is lichen sclerosis et atrophicus—or LSA. This is a relatively uncommon condition seen mainly in women in whom well defined patches of superficial atrophy of the epidermis occur with a white colour. There is fibrosis of the underlying tissues. It frequently occurs in the vulva and perineum and may also appear on the penis as balanitis xerotica obliterans. Extragenital lesions may occur anywhere on the skin. It may occur in a more acute form in children where it tends to resolve, but in adults it is a very chronic condition. There is an increased incidence of squamous cell carcinoma. Treatment is with topical steroids and excision of any areas that appear to be developing tumours.

The cause of the hyalinized collagen and epidermal atrophy is unknown, but in early lesions there is an infiltrate of lymphocytes with CD3, CD4, CD8, and CD68 markers. There is also an increase in Langerhans cells, so there may well be an immunological basis for these changes.

Vascular changes

Vascular lesions are associated with a wide range of conditions including infections, neoplasia, and allergic reactions. *Hormones*, particularly oestrogen, may affect the small blood vessels of the skin to produce telangiectasia and small angiomas, such as spider naevi.

Vasculitis and purpura, described in chapter 7, may be associated with disease of the kidneys and other organs. "Splinter haemorrhages" under the nails are usually the result of minor trauma but may be associated with a wide range of conditions, including subacute bacterial endocarditis and rheumatoid arthritis.

Livedo reticularis is a cyanotic, net-like discoloration of the skin over the legs. It may be idiopathic or associated with arteritis or changes in blood viscosity.

Erythrocyanosis is a dusky, red, cyanotic change in the skin over the legs and thighs, where there is a deep layer of underlying fat. The condition becomes worse in the winter months. It is most common in young women and usually resolves over the years. Lupus erythematosus, sarcoidosis, and tuberculous infection may localise in affected areas.

Telangiectasia and clubbing may be features of scleroderma in the CREST syndrome described above.

In *carcinoid* and *phaeochromocytoma* vasoactive substances cause episodes of flushing and telangiectasia.

CREST syndrome
- C—Calcinosis cutis
- R—Raynaud's phenomenon
- E—Esophagus
- S—Scleroderma
- T—Telangiectasia

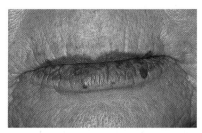
CREST syndrome

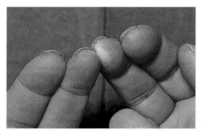
Calcinosis cutis

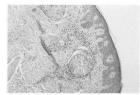
Vasculitis

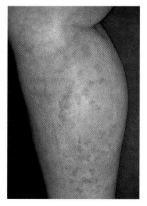
Livedo reticulosis

In *hereditary haemorrhagic telangiectasia* thin walled ectatic blood vessels develop in the mucous membranes and the skin—generally on the upper half of the body and the nail beds.

Erythemas

Erythema is macular redness of the skin due to congestion in the capillaries. It occurs as part of immunological reactions in the skin as in drug allergies and specific patterns of viral infections, such as measles. There are other types that show a specific pattern but are associated with a wide range of underlying conditions, such as erythema multiforme.

Erythema multiforme is associated with herpes and other viral infections or streptococcal and various bacterial infections, but also with many other conditions, particularly connective tissue disease, sarcoidosis, and reactions to drugs such as sulphonamides.

The lesions consist of erythematous macules becoming raised and typically developing into "target lesions" in which there is a dusky red or purpuric centre with a pale indurated zone surrounded by an outer ring of erythema. The lesions may be few or multiple and diffuse, often involving the hands, feet, elbows, and knees. Blisters may develop.

In the more severe forms there may be dermal changes and blister formation with involvement of the mucous membranes (*Stevens–Johnson syndrome*). There is often pyrexia with gastrointestinal and renal lesions. It can progress to *toxic epidermal necrolysis*, which some consider a form of erythema multiforme.

Erythema annulare is a specific pattern in the skin with a large number of reported associations, ranging from fungal and viral infections to sarcoidosis and carcinoma. It consists of a small erythematous macule that enlarges to form an expanding ring, usually on the trunk.

Erythema chronicum migrans is associated with *Borrelia* infection and Lyme disease—it is described on page 106.

There are many other types of "figurate erythemas". *Erythema gyratum repens* is associated with underlying carcinoma and *erythema marginatum*, which is now rare, with rheumatic fever.

Angiomas

Spider naevi, which show a central blood vessel with radiating branches, are frequently seen in women (especially during pregnancy) and children. If they occur in large numbers, particularly in men, they may indicate liver failure. Palmar erythema and yellow nails may also be present.

Congenital angiomas

Eruptive angiomas may be associated with systemic angiomas of the liver, lung, and brain. Port wine stain due to abnormality of the dermal capillaries commonly develops on the head and neck. It may be associated with congenital vascular abnormalities of the meningies and epilepsy. Vascular abnormalities of the eye, and also glaucoma, occur with lesions on the face.

Erythema of the nailbeds

This may be associated with connective tissue disease, such as lupus erythematosus, scleroderma, and dermatomyositis.

Changes in pigmentation

Hypopigmentation

Hormonal

A widespread partial loss of melanocyte functions with loss of skin colour is seen in hypopituitarism and is caused by an absence of melanocyte stimulating hormone.

Erythemas associated with systemic conditions
• Erythema multiforme
• Erythema annulare
• Erythema chronicum migrans
• Erythema gyratum repens
• Erythema marginatum

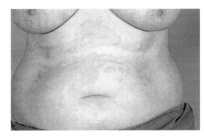

Figurate erythema

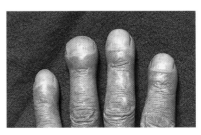

Erythema of nailbeds and clubbing

Genetic

In albinism, an autorecessive condition, there is little or no production of melanin with loss of pigment from the skin, hair, and eyes. Other genetic conditions with loss of skin pigment include piebaldism, phenylketonuria, and tuberous sclerosis.

Localised depigmentation is most commonly seen in vitiligo, in which a family history of the condition is found in one third of the patients. In the sharply demarcated, symmetrical macular lesions there is loss of melanocytes and melanin. There is an increased incidence of organ specific antibodies and their associated diseases.

Other causes of hypopigmented macules include: postinflammatory conditions after psoriasis, eczema, lichen planus, and lupus erythematosus; infections, for example, tinea versicolor and leprosy; chemicals, such as hydroquinones, hydroxychloroquine, and arsenicals, reactions to pigmented naevi, seen in halo naevus; and genetic diseases, such as tuberous sclerosis ("ash leaf" macules).

Hyperpigmentation

There is wide variation in the pattern of normal pigmentation as a result of heredity and exposure to the sun. Darkening of the skin may be due to an increase in the normal pigment melanin or to the deposition of bile salts in liver disease, iron salts (haemochromatosis), drugs, or metallic salts from ingestion. In agyria ingested silver salts are deposited in the skin.

Causes of hyperpigmentation include the following factors.

Hormonal

An increase in circulating hormones that have melanocyte stimulating activity occurs in hyperthyroidism, Addison's disease, and acromegaly. In women who are pregnant or taking oral contraceptives there may be an increase in melanocytic pigmentation of the face. This is known as melasma (or chloasma) and occurs mainly on the forehead and cheeks. It may fade slowly. Sometimes a premenstrual darkening of the face occurs.

Increased deposition of haemosiderin is generalised in haemochromatosis. Localised red-brown discoloration of the legs is seen with longstanding varicose veins. It also occurs in a specific localised pattern in Schamberg's disease, when there is a "cayenne pepper" appearance of the legs and thighs.

Neoplasia

Lymphomas may be associated with increased pigmentation. Acanthosis nigricans, characterised by darkening and thickening of the skin of the axillae, neck, nipples, and umbilicus, occurs with internal cancers, usually adenocarcinoma of the stomach. It is also seen in acromegaly. There is a benign juvenile type. Pseudoacanthosis nigricans is much more common, consisting of simple darkening of the skin in the flexures of obese individuals; it is not associated with malignancy.

Autoimmune associations with vitiligo	
• Thyroid disease	• Myasthenia gravis
• Pernicious anaemia	• Alopecia areata
• Hypoparathyroidism	• Halo naevus
• Addison's disease	• Morphoea and
• Diabetes	lichen sclerosus

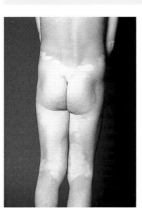
Vitiligo

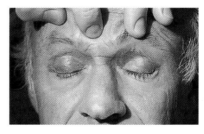
Agyria (silver salts in skin)

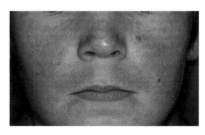
Melasma

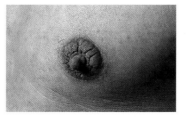
Acanthosis nigricans

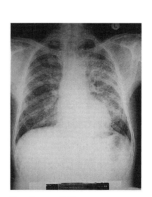
Carcinoma left upper zone

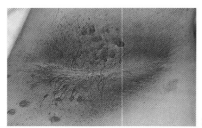
Pseudoacanthosis nigricans

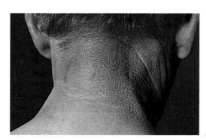
Acanthosis nigricans

Drugs

Chlorpromazine, other phenothiazines, and minocycline may cause an increased pigmentation in areas exposed to the sun. Phenytoin can cause local hyperpigmentation of the face and neck.

Inflammatory reactions

Postinflammatory pigmentation is common, often after acute eczema, fixed drug eruptions, or lichen planus. Areas of lichenification from rubbing the skin are usually darkened.

Malabsorption and deficiency states

In malabsorption syndromes, pellagra, and scurvy there is commonly increased skin pigmentation.

Congenital conditions

There is clearly a marked variation in pigmentation and in the number of freckles in normal individuals. There may be localised well defined pigmented areas in neurofibromatosis with "cafe au lait" patches. Increased pigmentation with a blue tinge occurs over the lumbosacral region in the condition known as Mongolian blue spot.

Peutz–Jeghers syndrome is described under the section "The gut and the skin", below. There are pigmented macules associated with intestinal polyposis in the oral mucosa, lips, and face.

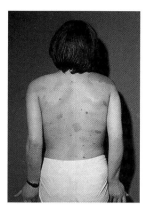

Neurofibromatosis

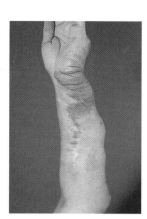

Neurofibromatosis

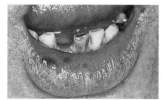

Increased pigmentation in malabsorption syndrome

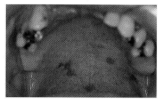

Peutz–Jeghers syndrome

Malignant lesions

Malignant lesions may cause skin changes such as acanthosis nigricans and dermatomyositis or produce secondary deposits. Lymphomas can arise in or invade the skin. Pruritus may be associated with Hodgkin's disease.

Mycosis fungoides is a T cell lymphoma of cutaneous origin. Initially well demarcated erythematous plaques develop on covered areas with intense itching. In many cases there is a gradual progression to infiltrated lesions, nodules, and ulceration. In others the tumour may occur de novo or be preceded by generalised erythema.

Poikiloderma, in which there is telangiectasia, reticulate pigmentation, atrophy, and loss of pigment, may precede mycosis fungoides, but it is also seen after radiotherapy and in connective tissue diseases.

Parapsoriasis is a term used for well defined maculopapular erythematous lesions that occur in middle and old age. Some cases undoubtedly develop into mycosis fungoides and a biopsy specimen should be taken of any such fixed plaques that do not clear with topical steroids.

Skin markers of internal malignancy

- Acanthosis nigricans—usually intra-abdominal lesions
- Erythematous rashes, "figurate erythema"
- Pruritus—usually lymphoma
- Dermatomyositis in the middle aged and elderly
- Acquired ichthyosis

Non-specific skin changes associated with malignant disease

- Secondary deposits
- Secondary hormonal effects
    Acne (adrenal tumours)
    Flushing (carcinoid)
    Pigmentation
- Generalised pruritus (particularly lymphoma)
- Figurate erythema
- Superficial thrombophlebitis
- Various eruptive skin lesions seen in Gardener's and Bazex syndromes

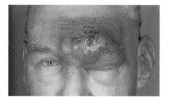

Lymphoma

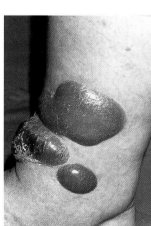

B cell lymphoma

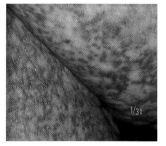

Poikiloderma

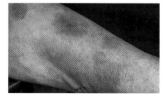

Parapsoriasis

The gut and the skin

Vasculitis of various kinds, periarteritis nodosa, connective tissue diseases such as scleroderma, and many metabolic diseases produce both cutaneous and gastrointestinal lesions. There are, however, some specific associations.

Dry skin, asteatosis, and *itching*, with superficial eczematous changes and a "crazy paving" pattern, occur in malabsorption and cachectic states. Increased pigmentation, brittle hair and nails may also be associated.

Pyoderma gangrenosum gives rise to an area of non-specific inflammation and pustules break down to form a necrotic ulcer with hypertrophic margins. There is an underlying vasculitis. There is a strong association with ulcerative colitis and also with Crohn's disease, rheumatoid arthritis, abnormal gamma globulins, and leukaemia.

Dermatitis herpetiformis, which has already been discussed, is an intensely itching, chronic disorder with erythematous and blistering lesions on the trunk and limbs. It is more common in men than women. Most patients have a gluten sensitive enteropathy with some degree of villus atrophy. There is an associated risk of small bowel lymphoma.

Peutz–Jeghers syndrome is inherited as an autosomal dominant characterised by the appearance in infancy of pigmented macules of the oral mucosal membranes, lips, and face. Benign intestinal polyps, mainly in the ileum and jejunum, which rarely become malignant, are associated with the condition.

Other conditions include congenital disorders with connective tissue and vascular abnormalities that affect the gut, such as Ehlers–Danlos syndrome and pseudoxanthoma elasticum (arterial gastrointestinal bleeding), purpuric vasculitis (bleeding from gastrointestinal lesions), and neurofibromatosis (intestinal neurofibromas).

In *Crohn's disease* (regional ileitis) perianal lesions and sinus formation in the abdominal wall often occur. Glossitis and thickening of the lips and oral mucosa and vasculitis may be associated.

Liver disease may affect the skin, hair, and nails to a variable degree. Obstructive jaundice is often associated with itching which is thought to be due to the deposition of bile salts in the skin. Evidence of this is the fact that drugs which combine with bile salts such as cholestyramine improve pruritus in some patients. Jaundice is the physical manifestation of bile salts in the skin.

Liver failure is characterised by a number of skin signs, particularly vascular changes causing multiple spider naevi and palmar erythema due to diffuse telangiectasia. It is not unusual to see spider naevi on the trunk in women but large numbers in men should raise suspicion of underlying hepatic disease.

Porphyria cutanea tarda as a result of chronic liver disease produces bullae, scarring, and hyperpigmentation in sun exposed areas of the skin. *Xanthomas* may be associated with primary biliary cirrhosis and in chronic liver disease asteotosis, with dry skin producing a "crazy paving" pattern.

Diseases that pyoderma gangrenosum may occur with
• Ulcerative colitis • Crohn's disease • Rheumatoid arthritis • Monoclonal gammopathy • Leukaemia

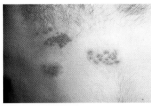
Early pyoderma gangrenosum

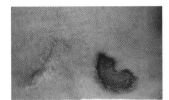
Pyoderma gangrenosum

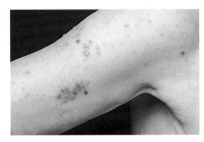
Dermatitis herpetiformis

Liver disease and the skin
Obstructive • Jaundice • Pruritus **Liver failure** • Multiple spider naevi (in men) • Palmar erythema • White nails—hypoalbuminaemia • Porphyria cutanea tarda **Cirrhosis** • Xanthomas (primary biliary cirrhosis) • Asteatosis

Diabetes and the skin

In diabetes the disturbances of carbohydrate–lipid metabolism, small blood vessel lesions, and neural involvement may be associated with skin lesions. The more common of these include the following.

Infection
Diabetic patients have an increased susceptibility to staphylococcal, coliform, and pseudomonal infection. *Candida albicans* infection is also more common in diabetics.

Vascular lesions
"Diabetic dermopathy", due to a microangiopathy, consists of erythematous papules which slowly resolve to leave a scaling macule on the limbs. Atherosclerosis with impaired peripheral circulation is often associated with diabetes. Ulceration due to neuropathy (trophic ulcers) or impaired blood supply may occur, particularly on the feet.

Specific skin lesions
Necrobiosis lipoidica
Between 40% and 60% of patients with this condition may develop diabetes, but it is not very common in diabetic patients (0·3%). As the name indicates, there is necrosis of the connective tissue with lymphocytic and granulomatous infiltrate. There is replacement of degenerating collagen fibres with lipid material. It usually occurs over the shin but may appear at any site.

Granuloma annulare
This usually presents with localised papular lesions on the hands and feet but may occur elsewhere. The lesions may be partly or wholly annular and may be single or multiple. There is some degree of necrobiosis, with histiocytes forming "palisades" as well as giant cells and lymphocytes. It is seen more commonly in women, usually those aged under 30. There is an association with insulin dependent diabetes. In itself it is a harmless and self limiting condition that slowly clears but may recur.

Other diseases

Porphyrias are due to the accumulation of intermediate metabolites in the metabolic pathway of haem synthesis. There are several types. In hepatic porphyrias there is skin fragility leading to blisters from exposure to the sun or minor trauma. In erythropoietic and erythrohepatic photoporphyrias there is intense photosensitivity. They are sometimes associated with sensitivity to long wavelength ultraviolet light that penetrates window glass.

Porphyria cutanea tarda usually occurs in men, with a genetic predisposition, who have liver damage as a result of an excessive intake of alcohol. There is impaired porphyria metabolism leading to skin fragility and photosensitivity, with blisters and erosions, photosensitivity on the face and the dorsal surface of the hands.

Xanthomas are due to the deposition of fat in connective tissue cells. They are commonly associated with hyperlipidaemia—either primary or secondary to diabetes, the nephrotic syndrome, hypothyroidism, or primary biliary cirrhosis. Four of the primary types are associated with an increased risk of atherosclerosis; type I is not. Diabetes may be associated with the eruptive type.

Necrotising fasciitis is an area of cellulitis that develops vesicles. Necrosis of the skin may indicate much more extensive, life threatening necrosis of the deeper tissues. Urgent surgical debridement is indicated.

Amyloid deposits in the skin occur in primary systemic amyloidosis and myeloma.

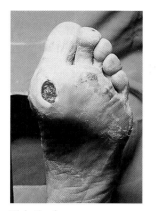
Diabetic ulcer

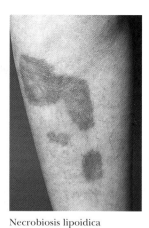
Necrobiosis lipoidica

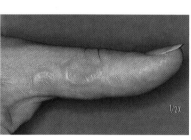
Granuloma annulare

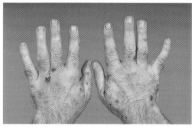
Porphyria

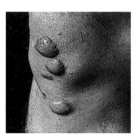
Xanthomas

Common types of xanthoma

Clinical type	Association with hyperlipidaemia Primary	Secondary
Xanthelasma of the eyelids—yellow plaques	II (may be normal)	
Tuberous nodules on elbows and knees	II, III	+
Eruptive—small yellow papules on buttocks and shoulders	I, III, IV, V	+
Plane—yellow macules, palmar creases involved	I, III	+
Generalised—widespread macules		myeloma
Tendons—swelling on fingers or ankles	II, III	+

Pregnancy

Pregnancy may be associated with pruritus, in which the skin appears normal in 15–20% of women (prunigo gestationis). It is generally more severe in the first trimester.

Polymorphic eruptions also present with pruritis with urticaria papules and plaques (the PUPP syndrome). It usually occurs on the abdomen in the third trimester and then becomes widespread. There may be a postpartum flare up. It can be a distressing condition for the mother but the baby is not affected, and it rarely recurs in subsequent pregnancies. Topical steroids can be used, but systemic steroids should be avoided.

Pemphigoid gestationis is a rare disorder that may resemble PUPP initially but develops pemphigoid-like vesicles, spreading over the abdomen and thighs: autoantibodies to the basement membrane are present.

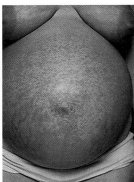
Polymorphic eruption

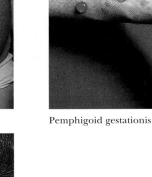
Pemphigoid gestationis

Sarcoidosis

Pulmonary and other systemic manifestation of sarcoidosis may occur without involvement of the skin. The most common changes are:

- Erythema nodosum, which is often a feature of early pulmonary disease.
- Papules, nodules, and plaques are associated with acute and subacute forms of the disease.
- Scar sarcoidosis, with papules occurring in scars.
- Lupus pernio is characterised by dusky red infiltrated lesions on the nose and fingers.

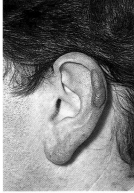
Nodule in sarcoidosis

Thyroid disease

Thyroid disease is associated with changes in the skin, which may sometimes be the first clinical signs. There may be evidence of the effect of altered concentrations of thyroxine on the skin, with changes in texture and hair growth. Associated increases in thyroid stimulating hormone concentration may lead to pretibial myxoedema. In autoimmune thyroid disease vitiligo and other autoimmune conditions may be present.

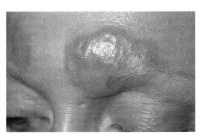
Sarcoid granuloma

Genetics and skin disease
by JA Savin

Though many genetic disorders of the skin are inherited in a classically Mendelian way (single gene disorders), others are genetically more complex. As a general rule, the common skin disorders that run in families, such as psoriasis, atopic eczema, and acne, tend to belong to the latter group.

Single gene disorders
Recent advances in genetic technology have been relatively easy to apply to these, usually rather uncommon, disorders, most of which had already been classified accurately on clinical grounds. Several things followed from this:

(1) The next step has often been an improvement in current clinical classifications, which can now be based logically on the underlying molecular abnormalities of the disorders in question. A good example of this is the modern classification of the inherited mechano-bullous disorders (also known as epidermolysis bullosa).

(2) New skin constituents were quickly recognized, their function being understood after studying the disorders in which they

Clinical signs of thyroid disease	
Hypothyroidism	**Hyperthyroidism**
Dry skin	Soft, thickened skin
Oedema of eyelids and hands	Pretibial myxoedema
Absence of sweating	Increased sweating (palms and soles)
Coarse, thin hair—loss of pubic, axillary, and eyebrow hair	Thinning of scalp hair
Pale "ivory" skin	Diffuse pigmentation
Brittle poorly growing nails	Rapidly growing nails
Purpura, bruising, and telangiectasia	Palmar erythema Facial flushing

are abnormal. Soon it was realized that the same molecules could be the targets both for genetic abnormalities and for acquired skin diseases. One example of this is the way in which autoantibodies directed against one of the constituents of hemidesmosomes (BP180) cause pemphigoid, whereas mutations in the gene responsible for BP180 are the basis of the junctional type of epidermolysis bullosa.

(3) Advances have been made too in our understanding of the structure and function of normal skin and its appendages—for example, the finding that melanocortin-1 receptor gene variants are associated with fair skin, red hair, and skin tumours.

(4) Mosaics were soon recognized. Clinically these are linear abnormalities in the skin, usually present at birth, which often contain cells with the same genetic abnormalities as those of known generalised genodermatoses. A good example of this is the way the same abnormalities in the genes controlling the production of keratins 1 and 10 can be responsible both for a generalised skin condition (epidermolytic hyperkeratosis) and for warty linear naevi. The mosaic areas follow Blashko's lines, a bizarre pattern of lines and whorls, which are not the same as dermatomes.

(5) The prenatal diagnosis of severe genodermatoses has become more accurate, though gene therapy has not yet fulfilled its early promise.

Genetically complex disorders

Psoriasis is a good example. It clusters in some families but does not follow a classical Mendelian pattern of inheritance. Environmental triggers are important, as well as genetic factors. Over the last few years, several wide scans of the genome have been undertaken with the aim of identifying the location of the genes that determine susceptibility to psoriasis. Five have been confirmed, all on different chromosomes, and now designated as Psors1 to Psors5. A further six loci may have similar effects, but the evidence for them is less strong. Psors1, on chromosome 6p21.3, is an especially important gene for psoriasis susceptibility in many populations and lies within the area of the major histocompatibility complex (MHC). However it is not itself an HLA class 1 gene, and may belong to the newly described MHC class 1 chain-related (MIC) gene family. The possession of one allele (A5.1) of this gene seems to lead to a type of psoriasis that starts especially early, and is more common in familial than in sporadic cases.

In *atopic eczema*, matters are equally complicated. Environmental factors may well be responsible for the recent rise in its prevalence as the gene pool within the population is not likely to have changed greatly, but a genetic component is obvious too, even though affected children can be born to clinically normal parents. Within each family, atopic disorders tend to run true to type, so that, in some, most affected members will have eczema, in others, respiratory allergy predominates. The inheritance of atopic eczema probably involves genes that predispose to the state of atopy, and others that determine whether it is asthma, eczema, or hay fever that develops. One plausible gene for the inheritance of atopy encodes for the β subunit of the high affinity IgE receptor, and lies on chromosome 11q13. However several groups have failed to confirm earlier reports of this linkage, and a gene linked to atopic eczema has recently been found on chromosome 3q21.

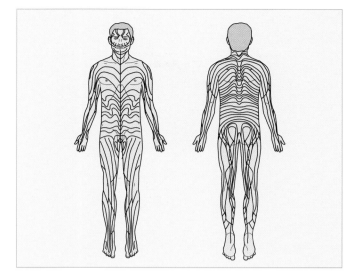

Blashko's lines

The abnormality underlying some inherited skin disorders

Skin disorder	Abnormality in
Ehlers–Danlos syndrome	Collagen and the extracellular matrix
Dystrophic epidermolysis bullosa	Type VII collagen
Pseudoxanthoma elasticum	Elastic tissue
Xeroderma pigmentosum	DNA repair
Simple epidermolysis bullosa	Keratins 5 and 14
Epidermolytic hyperkeratosis	Keratins 1 and 10
Palmoplantar keratoderma	Keratins 9 and 16
Junctional epidermolysis bullosa	Laminins
X-linked recessive ichthyosis	Steroid sulphatase
Darier's disease	Epidermal cell adhesion
Albinism (tyrosinase negative type)	Tyrosinase

Further reading

Fine JD, Eady RA, Bauer EA, et al. Revised classification system for inherited epidermolysis bullosa. *J Am Acad Dermatol* 2000;42: 1051–66

Harper J. *Inherited skin disorders.* Oxford: Butterworth–Heinemann 1999

Moss C, Savin JA. *Dermatology and the new genetics.* Oxford: Blackwell Science, 1995

17   Cutaneous immunology—Autoimmune disease and the skin

Types of allergic reaction

Allergic and other immune reactions may occur in the skin—the "immunological battleground of the body"—rather than involving internal organs. An acute vasculitis occurring in the skin is unpleasant and requires treatment but the same reaction occurring in the kidneys can be life threatening. The pattern of skin changes can indicate the type of immune process involved and also whether there is likely to be systemic involvement. The immune response of the skin is also used clinically in the tuberculin skin test to detect the level of immunity to tuberculosis. It is also the means of immunisation when an injection of inactivated organisms induces an immune response that protects the entire body.

The different types of immune reaction are all manifested in the skin as part of a normal response to pathogens or as an allergic reaction. The difference is expressed by the word "allergy", first used by Von Pirquet in 1906, derived from the Greek (αγοξ ενγον), meaning literally "other work". In other words it is a response that is appropriate for pathogenic organisms such as a tubercle bacillus but is misdirected against a harmless substance such as a rubber glove or the metal of a watch strap buckle.

Immunological reactions are of four types—five if autoimmunity is counted—of responses mediated by antibodies known as the humoral response and one by the lymphocytes known as the cell mediated response.

Immediate hypersensitivity

This type of reaction is caused by "reagin" antibodies, which consist mainly of lgE, that react with allergens such as housedust mite, animal dander, or grass pollens. These reactions may occur in both the skin or the lung to produce asthma. Allergic reactions to insect stings can cause severe systemic effects—"anaphylaxis", which literally means "without protection". Food proteins can also cause an immediate type of hypersensitivity reaction. The IgE molecule is attached to specific receptors on the surface of mast cells and when activated by linkage to specific allergen inflammatory mediators are released. This is an acute process, hence the name "immediate hypersensitivity".

The initial response occurring within five minutes is due to by the release of histamine, heparin, tryptophan. This is followed by inflammatory mediators—released in five to 30 minutes—leukotrien, prostaglandin. The later response, occurring after some hours, is caused by cytokines—predominantly tumour necrosis factor α (TNF-α) and interleukin 4 (IL4).

Severe reactions cause shock that is made worse by stress and exercise, as in the case of a young woman, allergic to wasp stings, who had a wasp sting when picnicking by a lake. She then plunged into the cold water, swimming vigorously, leading to a fatal anaphylactic reaction. Acute anaphylactic reactions to peanuts may be life threatening.

Cytotoxic reactions

In this case cells become the target of attack by circulating antibodies. There are a number of causes, such as drugs or proteins attached to the cell surface that act as haptens so they

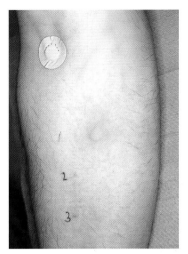

Reaction to fish protein

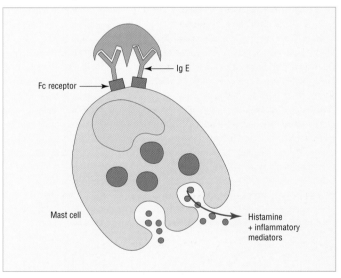

Type I—immediate hypersensitivity

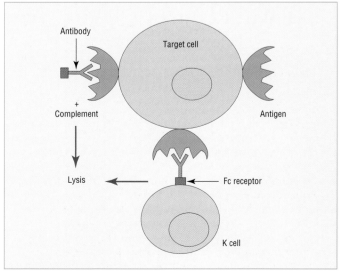

Type II—cytotoxic

become antigenic. This occurs in drug induced haemolysis from drugs. Alternatively, immune complexes are attached to the surface of the cell with the incorporation of complement leading to lysis. In haemolytic anaemia and incompatible blood transfusions antibodies are formed against erythrocytes. They may also be destroyed by killer cells. A typical example is haemolytic anaemia.

This immune response is the means of destroying cells that become antigenic as a result of being infected with virus.

In autoimmune diseases antibodies are directed against specific structures.

Antigen–antibody complex reactions
As a result of antibody production to antigens in the circulation, complexes form in the blood and these may be deposited in capillaries resulting in inflammatory changes. Similar changes may occur in the lung. This involves the activation of complement and the release of mediators of inflammation, producing vasodilatation and the accumulation of polymorphs.

Delayed hypersensitivity
This type of reaction results from lymphocytes known as T cells, because of their derivation from the thymus, which react with antigen in the skin. The reaction is initiated by antigen attached to Langerhan's cells in the epidermis being transported to the paracortical area of the regional lymph node with the production of lymphocytes sensitised specifically for that antigen. There is also the production of interleukin which has a feedback effect in stimulating the production of more sensitised lymphocytes.

The reaction of the T lymphocytes in the epidermis results in the accumulation of macrophages and the release of inflammatory mediators.

Autoimmune disease and the skin

DJ Gawkrodger

There is always the risk that the well developed human immune system may react against the body's own tissues, with a failure to distinguish between "self" and "non-self". An immune response develops which may be specific for a particular organ, such as the thyroid gland, or react against a number of different organs, as in connective tissue diseases. The skin can manifest both types of autoimmume response. The results of such reactions can be destruction of the cells concerned and the production of inflammation. There is an inherited tendency to autoimmune disease, marked by specific HLA (human lymphocyte antigen) in some cases.

The most common types of skin disease in which this autoimmune mechanism occurs are the blistering disorders, pemphigoid and pemphigus, as well as dermatitis herpetiformis.

Pemphigoid
In this condition large, tense blisters develop in which there are antibodies attached to the upper layer of the basement membrane at the dermo-epidermal junction, with an underlying inflammatory reaction producing a split above the basement membrane. Lysosomal enzymes are released damaging the basement membrane, resulting in separation of the epidermis and blister formation. The presence of

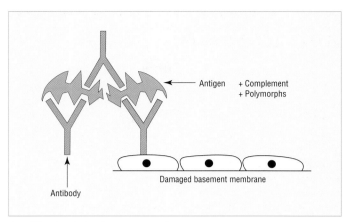

Type III—circulating immune complexes

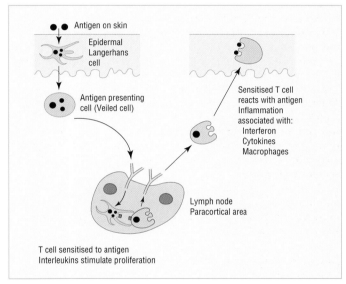

Type IV—delayed hypersensitivity

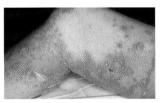

Reaction to metal

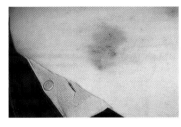

Blistering disorder as a result of an autoimmune response

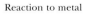

Split at dermo-epidermal junction

antibodies, usually IgG, can be shown by an antihuman IgG antibody labelled with fluorescein. When viewed under the microscope with ultraviolet light illumination, the presence of the IgG antibody is shown by fluorescence. The presence of circulating antibasement membrane antibodies in the serum can be shown either by direct immunofluorescence using a specimen of the patient's skin or by incubation by attachment to skin which has been incubated in serum from the patient.

The clinical features are described in chapter 8. The blisters develop, frequently with an erythematous background, on the limbs, trunk, and flexures. It is mainly seen in the elderly and is slightly more common in women.

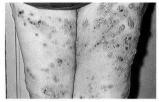

Direct immunofluorescence

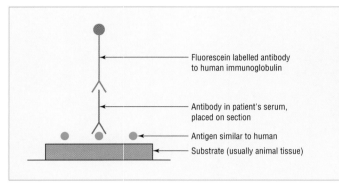

Indirect immunofluorescence

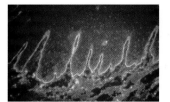

Indirect immunofluorescence

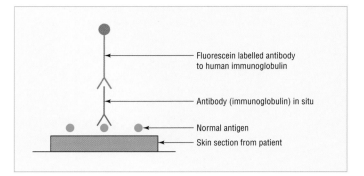

Indirect immunofluorescence   Pemphigus

Pemphigus

In this condition, antibodies are found to have developed against the epidermis above the basement membrane. The main antibody is IgG, but IgM and IgA may also be found. As a result of this reaction, there is separation of the epidermal cells with the formation of a superficial blister. A row of basal cells remains attached to the basement membrane. Direct immunofluorescence of the skin from affected patients shows that antibodies are deposited on the intercellular substance of the epidermis. Circulating antibodies are often present. Oral lesions are much more common than in pemphigoid.

Other organ-specific autoimmune diseases of the skin
Vitiligo
In this condition there is a loss of pigment as a result of antibodies developing against melanocytes in the skin in a limited area. However, the areas affected tend to gradually increase. There may be other autoimmune diseases in the same patient, causing, for example, pernicious anaemia, and thyroid disease.

Alopecia areata
There is evidence that this condition may be associated with an immune reaction against the hair follicle. The increased incidence of antibodies to the thyroid gland and gastric parietal cells in patients with alopecia areata provides circumstantial support for an autoimmune aetiology.

Non-organ-specific skin autoimmune disease
Systemic lupus erythematosus (SLE)
The hallmark of this condition is the presence of antibodies against various components of the cell nucleus. Although a wide range of organs may be affected, in three quarters of the patients the skin is involved, generally with an erythematous eruption occurring bilaterally on the face in a "butterfly" distribution. There may also be photosensitivity, hair loss, and areas of vasculitis in the skin. There is often intolerance of

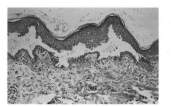

Intraepidermal split   Direct immunofluorescence

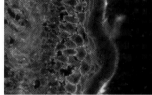

Range of autoimmune disease

Organ specific
- Hashimoto's thyroiditis
- Pernicious anaemia
- Addison's disease
- Myasthenia gravis
- Pemphigus
- Pemphigoid
- Vitiligo
- Primary biliary cirrhosis
- Rheumatoid arthritis
- Dermatomyositis
- Systemic sclerosis
Non-organ specific
- Lupus erythematosus

Range of autoimmune disease

Clinical variants of lupus erythematosus
- Systemic
- Subacute cutaneous
- Discoid
- (Neonatal)

sunlight. Subacute lupus erythmatosus is a variant that presents with an erythematous eruption in the skin and anticytoplasmic RNA molecules.

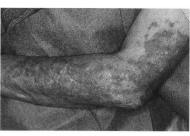

Subacute lupus erythematosus

Discoid lupus erythematosus (DLE)

This is a condition in which circulating antinuclear antibodies are very rare. There are quite well defined inflammatory lesions, with some degree of atrophy occurring on the face and occasionally on the arms as well.

Treatment of SLE with the threatened or actual involvement of organs is important. Prednisolone is usually required and sometimes immunosuppressant drugs such as azathioprine as well. Treatment of DLE is generally with topical steroids. Hydroxychloroquine by mouth is also used, generally in a dose of 200 mg daily. This drug can diminish visual acuity and this should be checked every few months. A simple chart, the Amsler Chart, is available for patients to use, consisting of a central dot with a grid which becomes blurred when held at arm's length when there is any impairment of acuity.

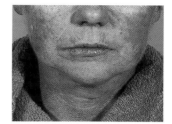

Subacute lupus erythematosus

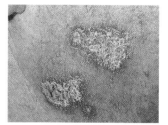

Discoid lupus erythematosus

Systemic sclerosis

This is a condition in which there is extensive sclerosis of the subcutaneous tissues in the fingers and toes as well as around the mouth (scleroderma), with similar changes affecting the internal organs, particularly the lung and kidneys. There are vascular changes producing Raynaud's phenomenon and telangiectasia around the mouth and fingers. It is associated with antinuclear antibodies (speckled or nucleolar), and in about 50% of cases circulating immune complexes may be present. Endothelial cell damage in the capillaries results in fibrosis and sclerosis of the organs concerned. There is considerable tethering of the skin on the fingers and toes, which becomes very tight with a waxy appearance and considerable limitation of movement. A variant is the CREST syndrome.

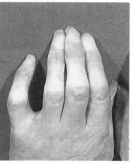

Systemic sclerosis

Morphoea is a benign form of localised systemic sclerosis in which there is localised sclerosis with very slight inflammation. There is atrophy of the overlying epidermis. The early changes often consisit of a dusky appearance to the skin.

The clinical features are described in chapter 16.

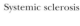
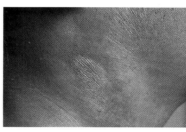

Morphoea

Dermatomyositis

This condition is described in chapter 16, but the main immunological features are deposition of IgG, IgM, and C3 at the dermo-epidermal junction in about half the cases in the early stages, as well as a lymphocytic infiltrate with CD4+ cells and macrophages. There are reports of autoantibodies in some patients. Dermatomyositis may represent an immune reaction to an underlying mechanism or derangement of the normal immune response.

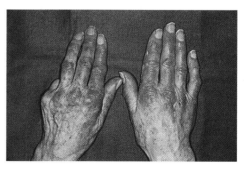

Dermatomyositis

Lichen sclerosus

This condition is also described in chapter 16 and is characterised by atrophic patches of skin. It occurs mainly in females and predominantly involves the genitals and perineum. The cause is unknown but in early lesions there is a band of lymphocytes, mainly CD3, CD4, and CD8. Immunoglobulins and complement accumulate in the affected areas. There is an association with vitiligo, morphoea, alopecia, and pernicious anaemia, suggesting an autoimmune association.

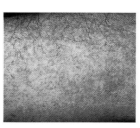

Lichen sclerosus

Graft versus host disease

This reaction occurs following bone marrow transplantation in immunosuppressed patients. T lymphocytes produced by the graft react against the body's own tissues, producing a skin eruption which may resemble measles. There is lysis of the basement membrane with shedding of the skin and sometimes lichen planus-like eruption. In the more chronic form, localised lesions develop, with immunoglobulins deposited in the walls of blood vessels with the activation of complement.

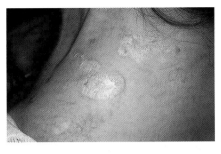

Graft versus host disease

Further reading

Roitt IM, Brostoff J, Male D. *Immunology*, 6th ed. St Louis: Mosby, 2001

18 Bacterial infection

RJ Hay

The process of infection involves the interaction between two organisms—the host and the invader. The clinical changes result from mechanisms involved in this process, notably the micro-organism, its virulence, and the patient's immune defenses. The lesions produced often have a well defined appearance, such as impetigo or tinea cruris, but the changes may be less specific.

Several features enable us to recognise that infection is a possible cause of the patient's condition. Acute bacterial infections generally produce some or all of the classical characteristics of acute inflammation.

> **Cardinal signs of infection**
> - Erythema
> - Swelling and oedema
> - Heat or warmth
> - Pain and discomfort

Erythema of the face

	Usually unilateral	Usually bilateral	Photosensitive
Acute			
(1) Allergic reactions			
Cosmetics		+	+ or −
Plants	+	or +	+ or −
Drugs		+	+ or −
(2) Urticaria		+	−
Reactions to light			
(3) Photodermatitis		+	+
Solar urticaria		+	+
(4) Infection			
Erysipelas		+	−
Fifth disease ("slapped cheek")		+	−
(5) Rosacea		+	+ or −
Chronic—recurrent			
(6) Lupus erythematosus			
Systemic		+	+
Discoid	+	or +	+
(7) Seborrhoeic dermatitis		+	−
(8) Acne		+	+
(9) Perioral dermatitis		+	−
(10) Vascular naevus	+	−	−

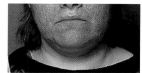
Allergic reactions to cosmetics

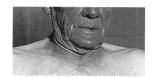
Photodermatitis

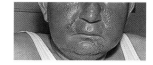
Erysipelas

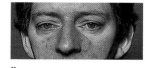
Rosacea

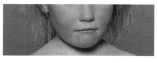
Fifth disease ("slapped cheek")

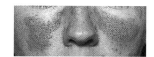
Systemic lupus erythematosus

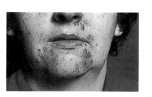
Perioral dermatitis

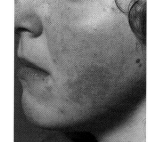
Vascular naevus

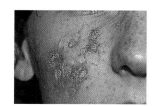
Discoid lupus erythematosus

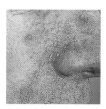
Seborrhoeic dermatitis

Clinical presentation

The woman shown in the photographs had acute *erysipelas* due to streptococcal infection, and all four features of inflammation were present. She was referred to the clinic with a diagnosis of an acute allergic response, which, from the appearance alone, was understandable. However, malaise and fever were also present and the lesions were warm and tender. The condition responded well to antibiotic treatment. The point of entry in such cases is thought to be a small erosion on the face. Erysipelas of the leg or foot may follow the development of a small fissure between the toes, but often there is no discernible portal of entry.

Erysipelas is the local manifestation of a Group A streptococcal infection, in the case illustrated the infection is confined to deep dermis as a form of cellulitis. However the same organism at distal sites, through the production of toxins or superantigens, can cause other skin lesions such as: (a) the rash of scarlet fever; (b) erythema nodosum; (c) guttate psoriasis; and (d) an acute generalised vasculitis.

Other forms of local bacterial infection include *impetigo*, *folliculitis*, and *furuncles* (boils). These conditions are caused by *Staphylococcus aureus* and in the case of folliculitis or boils the infection is associated with a local abscess. *Staph. aureus* colonises the anterior nares or perineum of normal people; it also commonly colonises eczema and may cause an acute exacerbation of atopic dermatitis.

Impetigo is a superficial infection of the skin of which there are two forms. In the non-bullous form the affected skin is covered with crusts. Both staphylococci and streptococci are responsible. However the bullous form which presents with blisters is due to staphylococci. Folliculitis, an inflammation of the hair follicle, is commonly caused by *Staph. aureus*. Infection of the scalp or beard hair (sycosis barbae) is uncommon but may become chronic. Abscess formation around the hair follicles may result in furuncles or boils; where several furuncles coalesce the lesion is known as a carbuncle.

Ecthyma, which is most common on the leg, is due to bacterial infection penetrating through the epidermis to the dermis causing a necrotic lesion with a superficial crust and surrounding inflammation. Both streptococci and staphylococci are responsible.

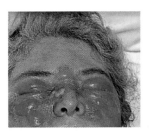

Acute erysipelas: presentation

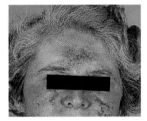

Acute erysipelas: patient shown in figure above two weeks later

Clinical presentation—points to note
- In any patient with a localised area of acute erythema, swelling, and fever—consider infection
- Remember that a generalised erythematous rash may be the manifestation of a localised infection. Scarlet fever arises from streptococcal sore throat, and herpes simplex of the lip may be associated with erythema multiforme
- The common pathogens are also commensals—recent studies showed that 69% of individuals are nasal carriers of *Staphylococcus aureus* and some may carry Group A streptococci in the throat

Mycobacterial disease

The clinical presentation of infections due to mycobacteria, a specific group of organisms that includes the causes of tuberculosis and leprosy, reflects the success of the host's response in eradicating organisms. There are clear differences, for instance, between disseminated miliary tuberculosis and lupus vulgaris or, for example, tuberculoid and lepromatous leprosy. These are discussed in chapter 23. As these infections are not common only lupus vulgaris and non-tuberculous or "atypical" mycobacterial infection are described.

Tuberculous mycobacterial infections
Lupus vulgaris presents as a very slowly growing indolent plaque. It usually represents a localised skin infection disseminated from a deep focus of infection. Squamous carcinomas may develop in long standing cases.

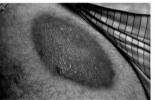

Lupus vulgaris

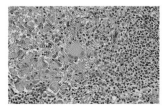

Mycobacterial disease—histology

Non-tuberculous mycobacterial infections

The most common is "fishtank" or "swimming pool" granuloma, acquired from tropical fish or rarely swimming pools, respectively, and caused by *Mycobacterium marinum*. Nodular lesions develop slowly with ulceration and may spread along local lymphatics to give a chain of nodules (sporotrichoid spread). Injection abscesses may be caused by mycobacteria such as *M. chelonei*. Buruli ulcer, an extensive ulcerating condition due to *M. ulcerans*, is confined to the tropics.

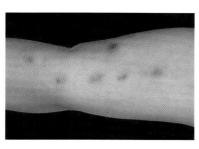
Swimming pool granuloma

Other infections

Rochalimea infections include bacillary angiomatosis, which presents in AIDS patients with small haemangioma-like papules, and cat scratch disease where crusted nodules appear at the site of the scratch associated with the development of regional lymphadenopathy one or two months later. A maculopapular eruption on the face and limbs or erythema multiforme may occur.

Psittacosis and ornithosis may be associated with a rash.

Rickettsial infections, including typhus, Rocky Mountain spotted fever, and rickettsial pox, are all associated with rashes, often purpuric.

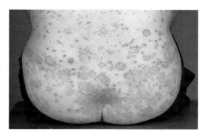
Secondary syphilis

Syphilis

There is a disseminated erythematous rash in secondary syphilis that is followed by a papulosquamous eruption, which affects the trunk, limbs, and mucous membranes. The palms and soles may be involved. There are also small clustered mouth ulcers. In patients with AIDS the rash of secondary syphilis is florid and often crusted or scaly.

Further reading

Carnwres O, Harman RM. *Clinical tropical dermatology*. 2nd ed. Oxford: Blackwell Scientific, 1992

Noble WC. *The skin: microflora and microbial skin disease*. Cambridge: Cambridge University Press

Common patterns of cutaneous bacterial infection

	Infected eczema	Impetigo (nonbullous)	Impetigo (bullous)
Appearance	Exudate Crusts Inflammation	Transient vesicles Exuding lesions with yellow crusts Erythema Affects mainly face and limbs, commonly in children	Erythema and bullae which rupture leaving superficial crusts Affects mainly face and limbs in children and adults
Cause	Persistent scratching Topical steroids	Toxic reaction between organisms and epidermis resulting in superficial epidermal split in bullous lesions	
Organisms	*Staphylococcus aureus* *Streptococcus pyogenes*	*Staphylococcus aureus* *Streptococcus pyogenes* in some outbreaks	*Staphylococcus aureus*
Treatment	(1) Weaker topical steroids (for the eczema) with topical antibiotics (2) Systemic antibiotics if necessary (3) Soaks with potassium permanganate	Topical antibiotics Systemic antibiotics against both streptococcal and staphylococcal infection	Topical and systemic antibiotics
Notes	• Avoid prolonged use of topical antibiotics • Return to using weaker steroid • It is wise to send a specimen for bacteriology: when infection has healed • Even without clinical evidence of infection most lesions of atopic eczema are colonised by *Staphylococcus aureus*	• Staphylococcal infection can cause generalised superficial shedding of the epidermis—"scalded skin syndrome" (Lyell's disease) • It is wise to send specimens for culture in an outbreak to identify presence of Group A streptococci potentially implicated in glomerulonephritis	

Boils (furuncles)	Folliculitis	Ecthyma	Erysipelas

Inflammatory nodule affecting the hair follicles develops into a pustule
Tender induration with severe inflammation, followed by necrosis
Heals with scarring
Affects all ages
Several boils may coalesce to form a carbuncle
	Various forms:
	(1) *Scalp*
	Children—"Follicular impetigo"
	Adults—
	  (a) Keloidal folliculitis Back of neck
	  (b) Acne necrotica Forehead/hairline
	(2) *Face*—"Sycosis barbae"
	(3) *Legs*—Chronic folliculitis
		Small bullae may be present initially
		An adherent crust is followed by a purulent ulcerated lesion with surrounding erythema and induration, which slowly heals
		Usually on legs
			Well defined areas of erythema—very tender, not oedematous
			Vesicles may form
			Common sites—abdominal wall in infants; in adults the lower leg and face
			An area of broken skin, forming a portal of entry, may be found

Underlying disease— for example, atopy Mechanical damage from clothing, occlusion	(1) Underlying disease— for example, eczema (2) Infection may be by mechanical precipitated injury, greasy emollients, and occlusive dressings	Hot climate, occlusion More common in debilitated individuals May follow secondary infection of chicken pox	Lymphoedema and severe inflammation due to bacterial toxins
Staphylococcus aureus, usually of same strain as in nose and perineum	*Staphylococcus aureus* *Propionibacterium acnes* *Malassezia* spp. *Pseudomonas* spp. and other Gram negative organisms	Both *Streptococci* and *Staph. aureus*	*Strep. pyogenes* (group A, but may be B, C, or G) *Staphylococcus aureus* *Klebsiella pneumoniae* *Haemophilus influenzae*
(1) Antibiotic (penicillinase resistant) systemically (2) Cleaning of skin with weak chlorhexedine solution or a similar preparation	Topical and long term systemic antibiotics— for example, erythromycin Topical antifungal for *Malassezia* infection	Improve nutrition Use antibiotic effective against both staphylococci and streptococci	Penicillin or erythromycin
• Nasal and perineal swabs should be taken to identify carriers • Remember unusual causes— a bricklayer presented with a boil on the arm with necrosis due to anthrax (malignant pustule) acquired from the packing straw used for the bricks	• Gram negative folliculitis occurs on the face—a complication of long term treatment for acne • Gram negative folliculitis on the body is associated with exposure to contaminated baths or whirlpools	• Check for debilitating diseases, reticuloses, diabetes	• Cellulitis affects the deeper tissues and has more diverse causes, being essentially inflammation of the connective tissue • *Streptococcus, Staphylococcus, Haemophilus*, and other organisms may be found • One of the complications of erysipelas of the face is thrombosis of the cavernous sinus

19   Viral infections

Like the pyogenic bacteria, viruses produce local lesions and may also cause a widespread reaction to the infection such as erythema multiforme. However, the clinical manifestations of common viral infections of the skin are easily recognised.

Local infective lesions caused by DNA viruses which can be isolated from the lesions themselves include the herpes and pox virus groups. In patients with AIDS chronic and widespread viral infections of the skin occur.

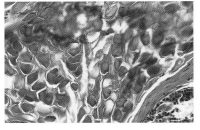

Molluscum inclusion bodies (a pox virus)

Herpes

Herpes simplex

The herpes simplex virus consists of two viral subtypes. Type I is associated with lesions on the face and fingers and sometimes genital lesions. Type II is associated almost entirely with genital infections. Recurrent episodes of infection are common, with both due to latent infection of sensory nerve ganglia.

Primary herpes simplex (type I) infection usually occurs in or around the mouth, with variable involvement of the face. Lesions are small vesicles which crust over and heal but there may be considerable malaise. Type II infection affects the external genitalia and waist area.

Recurrent infections are shorter lived (three to five days), occur in the distribution of a sensory nerve on the face or genitalia, and may be triggered by a variety of stimuli from sunlight to febrile illness.

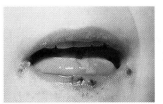

Herpes of lips

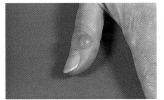

Inoculation herpes

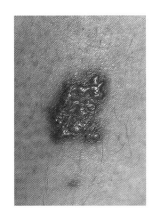

Herpes simplex

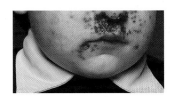

Eczema herpeticum

Herpes simplex—points to note

- The initial vesicular stage may not be seen in genital lesions, which present as painful ulcers or erosions
- There is usually a history of preceding itching and tenderness
- The most rapid methods of detecting virus from scrapings from the base of the ulcer are electronmicroscopy, immunofluorescence, or PCR
- Genital herpes in a pregnant woman carries a great risk of ophthalmic infection of the infant. Caesarean section may be indicated
- "Eczema herpeticum" or "Kaposi's varicelliform eruption" are terms applied to severe cutaneous and, less commonly, systemic, infection with herpes virus in patients with atopic eczema and some other skin conditions. Treatment is with oral or parenteral aciclovir

Herpes zoster

Varicella zoster virus (VZV) causes both chickenpox, the primary illness, and herpes zoster, which follows reactivation of the virus in the nerve ganglia. In zoster, pain, fever, and malaise may occur before erythematous papules develop in the area of the affected dermatome—most commonly in the thoracic area. Vesicles develop over several days, crusting over as they resolve. Secondary bacterial infection is common. Some patients develop episodes of pain in the affected area—postherpetic neuralgia after clearance of the rash. Skin lesions and nasopharyngeal secretions can transmit chickenpox.

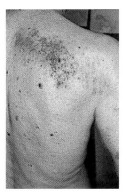

Herpes zoster

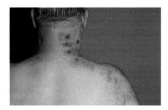

Herpes zoster

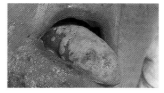

Mandibular zoster

Herpes zoster—points to note

- Trigeminal zoster may affect:
  the ophthalmic nerve (causing severe conjunctivitis)
  the maxillary nerve (causing vesicles on the uvula or tonsils)
  the mandibular nerve (causing vesicles on the floor of the mouth and on the tongue)
- Disseminated zoster is a severe illness presenting with widespread lesions. Visceral lesions may present with pleuritic or abdominal pain
- Extensive and haemorrhagic vesicles may develop in patients with AIDS

Treatment

Localised lesions of herpes simplex have been treated with a variety of medications from zinc sulphate to iodoxuridine. Topical acyclovir—a drug that inhibits herpes virus DNA polymerase—is effective but only shortens the duration of illness by a day or so. It is useful in primary infection but should be used as soon as the patient is aware of symptoms.

Severe, recurrent, herpes simplex, or herpes zoster can be treated with oral or intravenous aciclovir as early in the course of the illness as possible. Ganciclovir is an alternative.

Secondary infection may require antiseptic soaks, such as 1/1000 potassium permanganate, or topical or systemic antibiotics.

Steroids (prednisolone 40–60 mg/day) given during the acute stage of herpes zoster may diminish pain and postherpetic neuralgia.

Rest and analgesics are recommended treatment for extensive herpes simplex or herpes zoster infections.

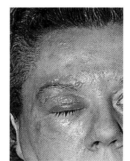

Ophthalmic zoster

Pox viruses

The pox viruses are large DNA viruses, with a predilection for the epidermis. Variola (smallpox), once a disease with high mortality, has been eliminated by vaccination with modified vaccinia (cowpox) virus.

Steroids may cause disseminated infection in immunodeficient patients

Molluscum contagiosum

The commonest skin infection due to a pox virus is molluscum contagiosum, a skin infection seen particularly in children. Despite its name it is not very contagious, but can occur in families.

In adults florid molluscum contagiosum may be an indication of underlying immunodeficiency, as in AIDS patients.

Clinical features

The white, umbilicated papules of molluscum contagiosum are characteristic. Large solitary lesions may cause confusion as can secondarily infected, excoriated lesions. These lesions often itch, particularly in patients with atopy. Resolving lesions may be surrounded by a small patch of eczema.

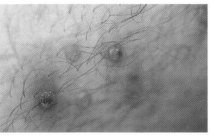

Molluscum contagiosum

Diagnosis

Diagnosis is usually based on clinical appearances or microscopy of the contents of papules. Sometimes there is confusion with viral warts.

Treatment

Most treatments result in discomfort and may not be tolerated by young children. An antibiotic–hydrocortisone ointment can be used for excoriated lesions. Treatment with liquid nitrogen is probably the simplest treatment. Other methods include superficial curettage and carefully rotating a sharpened orange stick moistened with phenol in the centre of each lesion.

Other pox virus infections

The other pox infections are of incidental interest.

Cowpox only sporadically infects cows from its natural reservoir, probably small mammals, and may affect humans. Papules on the hands enlarge and develop necrosis and crusting.

Milkers' nodules are due to a virus that causes superficial ulcers in cows' udders and calves' mouths. In humans papules form on the hands and develop into grey nodules with a necrotic centre, surrounding inflammation, and lymphangitis. A more generalised papular eruption can occur.

Orf is often recognised in rural areas. It is seen mainly in early spring as a result of contact with lambs. A single papule or group of lesions develops on the fingers or hands with purple papules developing into bulla. This ruptures to leave an annular lesion 1–3 cm in diameter with a necrotic centre. There is surrounding inflammation. The incubation period is a few days and the lesions last two to three weeks with spontaneous healing. Associated erythema multiforme and widespread rashes are occasionally seen.

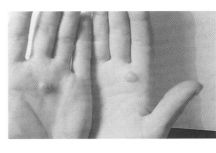
Cowpox, early stage

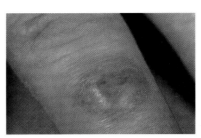
Milker's nodule

Wart viruses

A growing recognition that there is an association between human papilloma viruses (HPV), which cause warts, and cancer has led to a renewed interest in these infections. The wart is one of the few tumours in which a virus can be seen to proliferate in the cell nucleus. The different clinical forms of wart are caused by range of HPV, currently divided into over 80 major types. These viruses are also responsible for cervical cancer and have been associated with squamous carcinomas in the immunosuppressed. Warts are classed as cutaneous or mucocutaneous. Epidermodysplasia verruciformis is a rare condition associated with a defect of specific immunity to wart virus. The following aspects should be remembered:

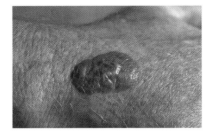
Orf

- Genital warts (due to HPV) very rarely undergo malignant change but HPV infection of the cervix, caused by type 16, frequently leads to dysplasia or in some cases malignant changes. Cervical smears must be taken.
- Very extensive proliferation of warts occurs in patients receiving immunosuppressive therapy, such as renal transplant recipients—in whom wart-like lesions can develop into squamous carcinomas—and in patients with AIDS.
- There is an association between HPV infections of the skin in immunosuppressed patients and the subsequent development of atypical-looking squamous carcinomas.
- Epidermodysplasia verruciformis, an unusual widespread eruption of flat erythematous warty plaques, can also develop into carcinoma.

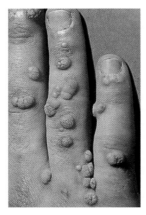
Common warts

Treatment

Warts commonly occur in children and resolve spontaneously without treatment or with very simple measures. These include paints or lotions containing salicylic and lactic acids in various proportions, which should be applied daily. Salicylic acid (40%) plasters are useful for plantar warts; they are cut to shape and held in place with sticking plaster for two or three days. Glutaraldehyde solution is also used.

For large or painful warts other measures can be used:

- Liquid nitrogen is effective but has to be stored in special containers and replaced frequently. It can be applied with cotton wool or discharged from a special spray with a focused nozzle. Freezing is continued until there is a rim of frozen tissue around the wart but not for more than 30 seconds. Subsequent blistering may occur. Scarring is unusual. Carbon dioxide is more readily available and can be transported in cylinders that produce solid carbon dioxide "snow". The temperature (about $-64\,°C$) is not as low as liquid N_2 ($-196\,°C$)
- Heat cautery causes more scarring and requires local anaesthesia. The diathermy loop is effective for perianal warts.
- Curettage and cautery together are effective but leave scars and the warts may recur.
- Podophyllin, 15–25% in tincture of benzoin compound or alcoholic solution, is effective for genital warts when applied each week. It is, however, toxic when ingested or absorbed, may cause burns, and must never be used in pregnancy.

Other treatments include laser therapy, immune enhancement (for example interferon β), and bleomycin injections. However, relapse is common whatever the remedy.

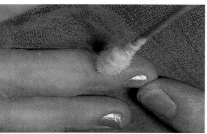
Treatment of warts with liquid nitrogen

Virus diseases with rashes

Measles and rubella are much less common than previously as a result of widespread immunisation. However, measles is probably the best known example of an exanthem (a fever characterised by a skin eruption. In an enanthem the mucous surfaces are affected.) Other common clinical patterns can then be compared with it. All exanthems, except fifth disease (erythema infectiosum), due to RNA viruses.

Virus diseases with rashes

- Measles
- Rubella
- Infectious mononucleosis
- Erythema infectiosum
- Roseola infantum
- Gianotti–Crosti syndrome
- Hand, foot, and mouth disease
- Primary HIV infection

Measles
- *Age.* Measles usually affects children, particularly those aged over five years.
- *Incubation* lasts seven to 14 days. Prodromal symptoms include: fever, malaise, upper respiratory symptoms; conjunctivitis; and photophobia.
- *Initial rash.* Early on Koplik's spots (white spots with surrounding erythema) appear on the oral mucosa. After two days a macular rash appears on the face, trunk, and limbs. Look behind the ears for early lesions.
- *Development and resolution.* The rash becomes papular, with coalescence. There may be haemorrhagic lesions and bullae which fade to leave brown patches.
- *Complications* are encephalitis, otitis media, and bronchopneumonia.
- *Diagnosis.* Specific antibodies may be detected; they are at their maximum at two to four weeks.

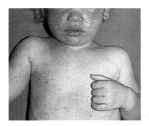
Measles

Rubella
- *Age.* Rubella affects children and young adults.
- *Incubation* lasts 14–21 days.
- *Prodromal symptoms.* There are none in young children. Otherwise fever, malaise, and upper respiratory symptoms occur.
- *Initial rash.* Initially some patients develop erythema of the soft palate and lymphadenopathy. Later pink macules appear on the face, spreading to trunk and limbs over one to two days.

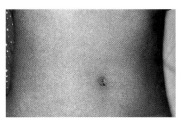
Rubella

- *Development and resolution.* The rash then clears over the next two days, and sometimes no rash develops at all.
- *Complications.* The most important complications are congenital defects in babies of women infected during pregnancy. The risk is greatest in the first month of pregnancy.
- *Diagnosis.* The diagnosis is made from the clinical signs above. Serum should be taken for antibodies and the test repeated at seven to 10 days.
- *Prophylaxis.* Active immunisation is routinely available for all schoolgirls.

Erythema infectiosum (fifth disease)
- *Age.* Erythema infectiosum affects children aged two to 10 years, mainly girls.
- *Incubation* lasts five to 20 days.
- *Prodromal symptoms.* There are usually none, but there may be a slight fever with initial rash.
- *Initial rash.* The initial rash is a hot, erythematous eruption on the cheeks—hence the "slapped cheek syndrome". Over two to four days a maculopapular eruption develops on the arms, legs, and trunk.
- *Development and resolution.* The rash extends to affect hands, feet, and mucous membranes, then fades over one to two weeks.
- *Diagnosis* is made by finding a specific IgM antibody to parvovirus B19.
- *Complications.* There are no reported dermatological complications but haematological disorders such as thrombocytopenia, arthropathy, and fetal abnormalities may be associated.

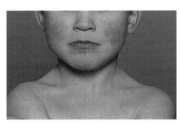
Erythema infectiosum

Roseola infantum
- *Age.* Roseola infantum affects infants aged under two years.
- *Incubation* lasts 10–15 days.
- *Prodromal symptoms.* There is fever for a few days.
- *Initial rash.* A rose pink maculopapular eruption appears on the neck and trunk.
- *Development and resolution.* The rash may affect the face and limbs before clearing over one to two days.
- *Diagnosis.* The condition is diagnosed from its clinical features.
- *Complications* include febrile convulsions.

Gianotti–Crosti syndrome
- *Age.* The Gianotti–Crosti syndrome affects children, usually those aged under 14 years.
- *Incubation* period is unknown.
- *Prodromal symptoms.* Lymphadenopathy and malaise accompany the eruption.
- *Initial rash.* Red papules rapidly develop on the face, neck, limbs, buttocks, palms, and soles.
- *Development and resolution.* Over two to three weeks the lesions become purpuric then slowly fade.
- *Diagnosis.* The syndrome may be due to a number of virus infections such as hepatitis B.
- *Complications.* Lymphadenopathy and hepatomegaly always occur and may persist for many months.

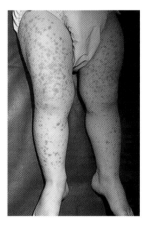
Gianotti–Crosti syndrome

Hand, foot, and mouth disease
- *Age.* Hand, foot, and mouth disease (Coxsackie virus A) affects both children and adults.
- *Incubation* period is unknown.
- *Prodromal symptoms.* Fever, headache, and malaise may accompany the rash.

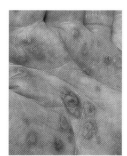
Hand, foot, and mouth disease

- *Initial rash.* Initially there may be intense erythema surrounding yellow-grey vesicles 1–1·5 mm in diameter. These are mainly distributed on the palms and soles and in the mouth. Sometimes a more generalised eruption may develop.
- *Development and resolution.* Over three to five days the rash fades.
- *Diagnosis.* Coxsackie A (usually A16) virus is isolated from lesions and stools. A specific antibody may be found in the serum.
- *Complications* are rare but include widespread vesicular rashes and erythema multiforme.

Other infections

Infectious mononucleosis

As well as the erythematous lesions on the palate a maculopapular rash affecting the face and limbs can occur.

Further reading

Joklik WK. *Virology*, 3rd ed. Norwalk: Appleton and Lange, 1988

Mandell GL, Douglas RG, Bennett JF. *Principles and practice of infectious diseases*, 3rd ed. New York: Churchill Livingstone, 1990

Timbury MC. *Notes on medical virology*, 9th ed. Edinburgh: Churchill Livingstone, 1991

White DO, Fenner FJ. *Medical virology*, 4th ed. New York: Academic Press, 1994

20   AIDS and the skin

MA Waugh

AIDS was first described in 1981 and since then 22 million people have died of the disease. The World Health Organisation estimates that in December 2000, 36 million people were infected with HIV. Of these, 1·5 million were children under the age of fifteen. It is estimated that 5·3 million people were newly infected with HIV in the year 2000 and 3 million have died in the same year. A total of nearly 22 million people have died of AIDS since the start of the epidemic. In the United Kingdom the prevalence of HIV infection is about 30 000. Over 65 000 in Europe are infected.

The human immunodeficiency virus (HIV) is the cause of the acquired immunodeficiency syndrome (AIDS). This virus was first isolated in 1983 in Paris and a second retrovirus, HIV2, was isolated from West Africa in 1986. The virus contains an enzyme that copies viral RNA into the DNA of the host cell in which the HIV virus then persists in the host cells, particularly monocytes, macrophages, and dendritic cells.

Skin lesions in patients with AIDS

- Skin lesions can develop as a manifestation of primary HIV infection
- Skin lesions can develop as a consequence of immunosuppression (AIDS)

Between these two events there is a latent period that can last from a few months to several years

---

Stages of AIDS

Primary HIV infection
In 80% of cases there are initial symptoms and signs—"seroconversion illness". There are a variety of symptoms including fever, malaise, headache, nausea, vomiting, and diarrhoea. There is often lymphadenopathy. The skin signs consist of a transient maculopapular eruption associated with erythema and erosions in the mouth in some patients.

Early stages
In the early stages 50% of patients have antibiotics to HIV and the p24 antigen can be detected. The proportion of CD4 lymphocytes decreases, and this is associated with the development of secondary changes in the skin. There is also an increase in HIV antibodies so a test for this should be repeated six to eight weeks after the initial illness. Counselling should take place before testing is carried out.

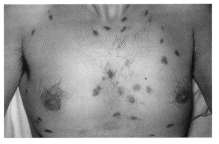

Flexural candidiasis

Late stage HIV disease
The skin changes are many and variable. Common inflammatory skin diseases such as psoriasis and seborrhoeic dermatitis will be much more florid. Cutaneous infections are more severe due to the impaired immune response and opportunistic infections also develop. In addition, Kaposi's sarcoma occurs in 34% of homosexual men and in 5% of other cases.

AIDS should therefore be considered in any patient with a florid inflammatory skin disease that is resistant to treatment or severe and extensive infection of the skin.

Kaposi's sarcoma

Skin changes in AIDS

Seborrhoeic eczema
This is common and may be the only evidence of HIV infection initially. It is more extensive and inflamed than usual. The role of *Pityrosporum* organisms is indicated by the response to imidazole antifungal drugs.

Psoriasis
Psoriasis is more widespread, severe, and resistant to treatment in patients with late HIV disease. The use of ultraviolet light may lead to an increased risk of Kaposi's sarcoma.

Infections
Any type of opportunistic infection is more likely in patients with AIDS and will generally be more severe. An itching, inflammatory folliculitis occurs in many cases. The cause is unknown, but it is possible that *Demodex* spp. play a part.

Fungal infections
Superficial fungal infections are often much more extensive and invade more deeply into the dermis than usual. There may also be granuloma formation.

Deep fungal infections that are not normally seen in healthy individuals occur in AIDS patients as opportunistic infections. *Cryptococcus neoformans* and *Histoplasma capsulatum* may cause inflammatory papular and necrotic lesions, particularly in the later stages of the disease.

Candidiasis is common and often associated with bacterial infections. It occurs particularly in and around the mouth, on the palate, and in the pharynx. It commonly causes severe vulvovaginitis in infected women.

Pityrosporum organisms occur more frequently and may produce widespread pityriasis versicolor on the trunk or extensive folliculitis.

Bacterial infections
Impetigo may be severe, with particularly large bullous lesions occurring.

Mycobacteria may produce widespread cutaneous and systemic lesions. Varieties of mycobacteria that do not normally infect the skin may cause persistent necrotic papules or ulcers.

Viral infections
Both herpes simplex and herpes zoster infections may be unusually extensive, with large individual lesions. In the case of herpes zoster the affected area may extend beyond individual dermatomes. Sometimes persisting ulcerated lesions occur.

Molluscum contagiosum lesions are frequently seen. They are much larger than usual and develop over quite large areas of skin. They are readily identified as small, firm papules with an umbilicated centre. When very large individual molluscum lesions occur they may be due to localised fungal infection, particularly cryptococcus and histoplasmosis.

Viral warts may be large and extensive. Perianal and genital warts due to the human papilloma virus (HPV) are common and may be associated with intraepithelial neoplasia of the cervix and sometimes invasive perianal squamous cell carcinoma. The warts tend to become smaller as the immune status of the patient improves with the treatment. It is not unusual for florid viral warts to develop in the mouth.

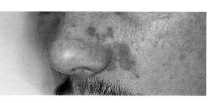
Seborrhoeic dermatitis

Skin changes in AIDS
- Seborrhoeic eczema
- Psoriasis
- Fungal infections
- Bacterial infections
- Viral infections
- Kaposi's sarcoma
- Drug rashes
- Oral hairy leukoplakia

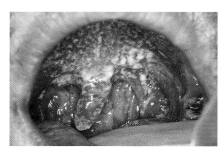
Pseudomembranous candida

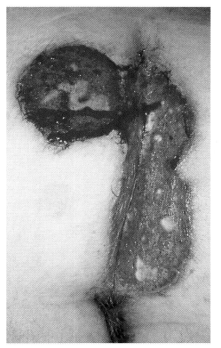
Aciclovir–resistant perianal herpes simplex infection

Other manifestions

Oral hairy leukoplakia occurs in 30–50% of patients with AIDS. It is characterised by an overgrowth of epithelial plaques on the sides of the tongue with a verrucous surface and a grey/white colour. It is believed to be due to a proliferation of the Epstein–Barr virus.

Infestations with various organisms is not uncommon and the severe widespread crusted lesions of Norwegian scabies may occur.

Kaposi's sarcoma

Kaposi's sarcoma is associated with the later stages of AIDS but can occur earlier. It is associated with herpes virus type 8. It often presents with small polychromic macules on the face, palate, trunk or groin which vary from red and purple to brown. They then develop into larger livid plaques, involving the trunk, limbs, and face, and also the oral mucosa. They are most common on the palate and nose. Sometimes the lesions are very aggressive.

B cell lymphoma may occur in the skin in 10% of AIDS patients. There is also an increased incidence of basal cell and squamous carcinomas.

Drug rashes

Reactions to sulphonamides and antibiotics are not uncommon, usually presenting as a maculopapular eruption. Occasionally this can be severe and associated with Stevens–Johnson syndrome. Myopathy may occur as a reaction to zidovudine.

All the above manifestions of AIDS become less marked as the CD4 count improves with treatment.

AIDS may thus present with a wide variety of skin conditions, commonly with several present at the same time. Any unusually florid skin condition that is resistant to treatment should raise the suspicion that HIV infection may be present.

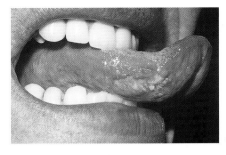

Oral hairy leukoplakia

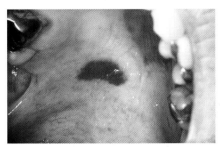

Kaposi's sarcoma of the hard palate

Further reading

Adler MW. *ABC of AIDS*, 4th ed. London: BMJ Publishing Group, 1997
Penneys NS. *Skin manifestations of AIDS*, 2nd ed. St Louis: Mosby, 1995

21   Fungal and yeast infections

RJ Hay

Fungal infections

The common fungal infections of the skin are dermatophytosis or "ringworm", superficial candidiasis, and *Malassezia* infections. There are two growth forms of fungi, moulds, and yeasts. Mould fungi produce thread-like hyphae that comprise chains of cells. In dermatophyte fungal infection of the skin, hair, and nails these hyphae invade keratin and are seen on microscopic examination of skin, hair, or nails from infected tissues. Vegetative spores (conidia) develop in culture, and their distinctive shape helps to identify the different species. Skin scrapings or clippings from infected nails can be easily taken and should always be sent to the laboratory for mycological examination and culture in any patient suspected of having a fungal infection.

In yeast infections such as those due to candida, the fungal cells are individual and separate after cell division by a process called budding. In systemic, or deep, fungal infections subcutaneous on deep visceral structures are attacked. However skin involvement can also occur following blood stream dissemination and such lesions may provide a clue to the diagnosis.

Why should one suspect a lesion to be due to a fungus?

Clinical presentation

Fungal infections usually itch. Those due to zoophilic (animal) fungi generally produce a more intense inflammatory response with deeper indurated lesions than fungal infections due to anthropophilic (human) species. Some lesions, usually those on the trunk, have a prominent scaling margin with apparent clearing in the centre. Hence the name "ringworm".

Children below the age of puberty are susceptible to scalp ringworm and anthropophilic fungi (from humans) have become common in some inner city areas. They can also be infected with zoophilic fungi (from animals), particularly cattle, dogs, and cats. Cattle ringworm can cause an intense inflammatory response in children, producing a "kerion" described below. They rarely develop anthropophilic fungal infection.

Adults. From adolescence onwards infection of the feet is a common occurrence. Tinea cruris in the groin is seen mainly in men and fungal nail infections (onychomycosis) have become particularly common.

Infection from dogs and cats with a zoophilic fungus (*Microsporum canis*) to which humans have little immunity can occur at any age. A patient returned from a skiing holiday with intensely itchy "eczema", which refused to clear. A stray kitten, mewing outside in the dark, had been taken indoors, warmed in their sleeping bags, and infected the whole party with *M. canis*.

Nail infections

These occur mainly in adults, usually in their toenails, especially when traumatised—for example the big toes of

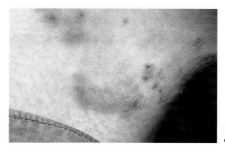

Tricophyton rubrum infection of the neck

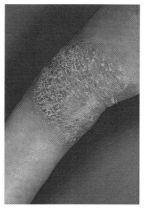

Animal ringworm

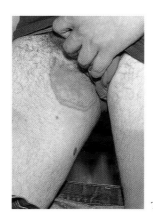

Tinea cruris

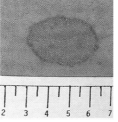

Microsporum canis

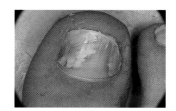

Fungal infection of nail

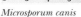

footballers. The nails become thickened and yellow and crumble, usually asymmetrically. The changes occur *distally* and move back to the nailfold. In psoriasis of the nail the changes occur *proximally* and tend to be symmetrical and are associated with pitting and other evidence of psoriasis elsewhere.

Chronic paronychia occurs in the fingers of individuals whose work demands repeated wetting of the hands: housewives, barmen, dentists, nurses, and mushroom growers, for example. Other predisposing factors include diabetes, poor peripheral circulation, and removal of the cuticle. There is erythema and swelling of the nail fold, often on one side with brownish discoloration of the nail. Pus may be exuded. The cause is *Candida albicans* (a yeast) together with secondary bacterial infection.

Pushing back the cuticles should be avoided—this is commonly a long term condition, lasting for years. The hands should be kept as dry as possible, an azole lotion applied regularly around the nail fold, and in acute flares a course of erythromycin prescribed.

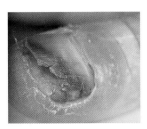

Chronic paronychia

Feet

Tinea pedis, or athletes foot, is a common disease and its prevalence increases with age. It is easily acquired in public swimming pools or showers and industrial workers appear to be particularly predisposed to this infection. The hands may be affected.

In interdigital tinea pedis the itching, macerated skin beneath the toes is familiar, but when a dry, scaling rash extends across the sole and dorsal surface of the foot (dry type tinea pedis) the diagnosis may be missed. The condition needs to be differentiated from psoriasis and eczema.

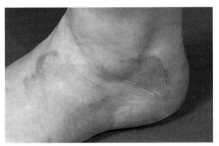

Tinea pedis

Hands

Dermatophyte infections often produce a dry rash on one palm. There may be a well defined lesion with a scaling edge.

Trunk

Tinea corporis presents with erythema and itching and a well defined scaling edge. In the groin, tinea cruris, the infection may spread to the adjacent skin on the thighs and abdomen. Intense erythema and satellite lesions suggest a candida infection. In the axillae erythrasma due to *Corynebacterium minutissimum* is more likely. It does not respond to antifungal treatment but clears with tetracycline by mouth.

Tinea versicolor affects the trunk, usually of fair skinned individuals exposed to the sun. It affects mainly the upper back, chest, and arms. Well defined macular lesions with fine scales develop, which tend to be white in suntanned areas and brown on pale skin. It may be confused with seborrhoeic dermatitis, pityriasis rosea, and vitiligo. In skin scrapings the causative

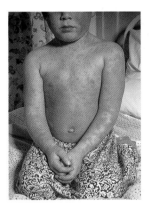

Tinea corporis

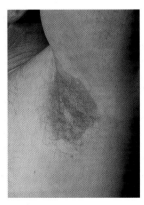

Erythrasma

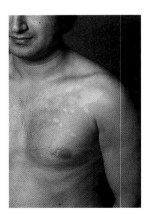

Tinea versicolor

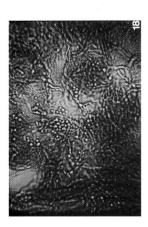

Pityrosporum organisms

organisms, *Malassezia* spp., normally found in hair follicles, can be readily seen.

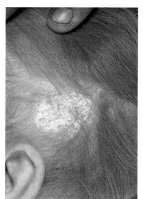
Microsporum ringworm

Scalp and face

Scalp ringworm in children may be caused by anthropophilic fungi such as *Trichophyton tonsurans*, which is spreading in cities in the United Kingdom, or *Microsporum audouinii*. Sporadic cases are caused by *M.canis* which is acquired from cats or dogs. In all cases there is itching, hair loss, and some degree of inflammation which is worse with *M. canis* infections.

Kerion, an inflamed, boggy, pustular lesion, is often due to cattle ringworm and is fairly common in rural areas. It is often seen in children in the autumn when the cows are brought inside for the winter.

Tinea incognito is the term used for unrecognised fungal infection in patients treated with steroids (topical or systemic). The normal response to infection (leading to erythema, scaling, a raised margin, and itching) is diminished, particularly with local steroid creams or ointments. The infecting organism flourishes, however, because of the host's impaired immune response—shown by the enlarging, persistent skin lesions. The groins, hands, and face are sites where this is most likely to occur.

Seborrhoeic dermatitis of adults may also be caused by *Malassezia*.

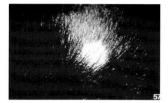
Microsporum—Wood's light

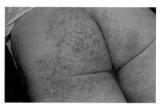
Tinea incognito

Yeast infections

Candida infection may occur in the flexures of infants and elderly or immobilised patients, especially below the breasts and folds of abdominal skin. It needs to be differentiated from: (a) psoriasis, which does not itch; (b) seborrhoeic dermatitis, a common cause of a flexural rash in infants; and (c) contact dermatitis and discoid eczema, which do not have the scaling margin. Candida intertrigo is symmetrical and "satellite" pustules or papules outside the outer rim of the rash are typical. Yeasts, including *Candida albicans*, may be found in the mouth and vagina of healthy individuals. Clinical lesions in the mouth—white buccal plaques or erythema—may develop. Predisposing factors include: general debility, impaired immunity (including AIDS), diabetes mellitus, endocrine disorders, such as Cushing's syndrome, and corticosteroid treatment. Vaginal candidosis or thrush is a common infection of healthy young women; an underlying predisposition is rarely found. The infection presents with itching, soreness, and a mild discharge.

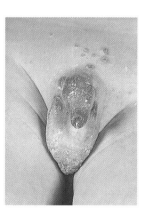
Candida albicans

Deep fungal infection

Fungal infections of the deeper tissues are only rarely associated with skin lesions in the United Kingdom, except in patients with AIDS. Some infections that involve deep tissue, histoplasmosis, cryptococcosis, and infections due to *Penicillium marneffei*, can present with skin lesions. In an HIV positive patient lesions resembling molluscum contagiosum may be the earliest feature of deep fungal infections.

In tropical countries deep fungal infections are more common. These are described in chapter 23. They should be considered in any patient from a tropical country with chronic indurated and ulcerating lesions.

Treatment

Topical treatment

The most commonly used treatments are the imidazole preparations, such as clotrimazole and miconazole (two to

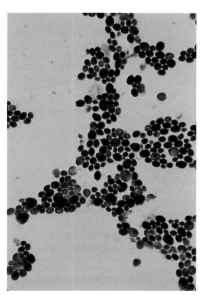
Candida organisms

four weeks) and also topical terbinafine (one to two weeks). The polyenes, nystatin, and amphotericin B are also effective against yeast infection. For damp macerated skin dusting powders may be helpful. In toe web infections a mixture of micro-organisms including dermatophytes and Gram negative bacteria may be present and both require treatment.

Systemic treatment

It is important to confirm the diagnosis from skin scrapings before starting treatment. Terbinafine is a very effective fungicidal drug. It is taken in a dosage of 250 mg once daily for two to six weeks for skin infections, six weeks for finger nail or three months for toenail infections. It is only approved for use in children in some countries. Blood monitoring is only advised in patients with liver disease or impaired renal function. Pregnancy and lactation are relative contraindications. There have been reports of headaches, taste disturbances and, very rarely, liver dysfunction.

Triazole preparations such as itraconazole are effective in both dermatophyte and yeast infections. Cases of liver damage have rarely been reported. Fluconazole is effective in yeast infections. Some drugs interact with azole drugs, the main ones being terfenadine, astemizole, digoxin, midazolam, cyclosporin, tacrolimus, and anticoagulants.

Griseofulvin is mainly used for tinea capitis. The duration of treatment is six to eight weeks for infections of the scalp. The dose is 10–20 mg/kg for children, taken with food. Contraindications to griseofulvin are severe liver disease and porphyrias. The drug interacts with the coumarin anticoagulants.

In countries without access to these drugs simple measures such as antiseptic paints—Neutral Red or Castellan's paint—can be used. Whitfield's ointment (benzoic acid ointment) is easily prepared and is reasonably effective for fungal infections.

Principles of diagnosis and treatment

- Consider a fungal infection in any patient where isolated, itching, dry, and scaling lesions occur without any apparent reason—for example, if there is no previous history of eczema. Lesions due to fungal infection are often asymmetrical
- Skin scrapings or clippings should be sent to the laboratory from lesions, nails, or hair. The skin scales should be removed by scraping the edge of the lesion with a scalpel held at right angles to the skin on to a piece of dark paper—transport packs are available commercially. Clippings can be taken from the nails and as much material as possible should be taken from the nail including subungual debris. Laboratories will report first on the direct microscopy of the material examined after treatment with 10% potassium hydroxide but culture results take at least two weeks
- Lesions to which steroids have been applied are often quite atypical because the normal inflammatory response is suppressed—*tinea incognito*. The patient often states that the treatment controls the itch but the rash persists and may change into a tender form of folliculitis. In such cases microscopy of lesions is usually strongly positive
- Wood's light (ultraviolet light filtered through special glass) can be used to show *Microsporum* infections of hair, as they produce a green-blue fluorescence

Further reading

Midgley G, Clayton Y, Hay RJ. *Medical mycology*. London and St Louis: Mosby-Wolfe, 1997

Elewski BE. *Cutaneous fungal infections*. New York: lgaku-Shoin, 1992

Evans EG, Richardson MD. *Medical mycology: A practical approach*. Oxford: Oxford University Press, 1989

22 Insect bites and infestations

So, naturalists observe, a flea
Hath smaller fleas that on him prey;
And these have smaller fleas to bite 'em.
And so proceeds "Ad infinitum"
                    Jonathan Swift

It is, of course, the internal parasites of biting insects that cause trouble for humans, rather than "smaller fleas" on their surface.

An ornithologist went bird watching in Guyana, where he sustained widespread "midge bites" on the arms. He was referred on account of nodules that developed a few weeks later, then enlarged and ulcerated. Other lesions occurred further up the arms with regional lymphadenopathy. A biopsy specimen showed histiocytic inflammatory changes, and *Leishmania braziliensis* was isolated from smears; the midges (phlebotomus or sand fly) had acquired the protozoon while feeding on local rodents and transferred it into the ornithologist's skin.

Serious disease from insect vectors is rare in residents of most Western countries but, as in the patient described above, must be considered in those returning from tropical and subtropical countries.

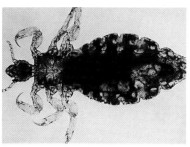
Body louse

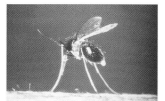
Sand fly

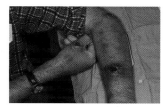
Leishmaniasis

Some diseases with skin lesions resulting from insect bites

Condition	Appearance	Organism	Vector
Cutaneous leishmaniasis	Chronic enlarging nodules with ulceration	Leishmania protozoon (*L. braziliensis*)	Sand fly
Oriental sore	Ulcerating nodules	Leishmania (*L. tropica*)	Sand fly
Kala-azar	Hypopigmented, erythematous, and nodular lesions	Leishmania (*L. donovani*)	Insect vectors
Onchocerciasis	Pruritic nodules	Filaria (*Onchocerca volvulus*)	Black fly (Simuliidae)
Typhus, human	Erythematous rash and systemic illness	Rickettsia (*R. prowazekii*)	Human louse
Typhus, murine		(*R. mooseri*)	Rat flea
Rocky Mountain spotted fever	Maculopapular rash and fever	Rickettsia (*R. rickettsii*)	Ticks
Rickettsial pox	Vesicular eruption like chickenpox	Rickettsia (*R. akari*)	House mouse, louse
Tick typhus	Necrotic lesions, maculopapular rash, and fever	Various rickettsias	Ticks
Scrub typhus	Fever, lymphadenopathy, maculopapular rash	Rickettsia (*R. tsutsugamushi*)	Mites
Relapsing fever	Widespread maculopapular lesions	*Borrelia recurrentis*	Lice, ticks
Lyme disease	May be annular	*Borrelia burgdorferi*	Ticks, black fly
Yellow fever and dengue	Flushing of face, scarlatiniform rash	Arbovirus	Aedes mosquito

Most cases of bites from fleas, midges, and mosquitoes are readily recognised and cause few symptoms apart from discomfort. Occasionally an allergic reaction confuses the picture, particularly the large bullae that can occur from bites on the arms and legs. It may be difficult to persuade patients that their recurrent itching spots are simply due to flea bites and the suggestion may be angrily rejected.

Nevertheless, some patients are convinced that they have an infestation when they do not. Often they will bring small packets containing "insects". Examination shows these to be small screws of wool, pickings of keratin, thread, and so on. Sympathy and tact will win patients' confidence; derision and disbelief will merely send them elsewhere for a further medical opinion. Antipsychotic drugs may help to dispel the delusion of parasitic infestation (delusional parasitosis) and should be used in conjunction with advice from a psychiatrist if possible. These drugs should be used with care and with full awareness of their side effects, particularly in patients with cardiovascular disease and a history of epilepsy. Pimozide has been used in the past but because of its side effects risperidone is preferred.

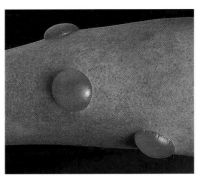

Bullae caused by insect bites

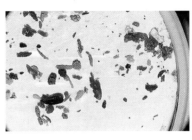

Parasitophobia specimens

- Flea bites, including those from *Cheyletiella* mites in dogs and cats, occur in clusters, often in areas of close contact with clothing, for example, around the waist.
- Grain mites (*Pyemotes*) and harvest mites (*Trombiculidae*) can cause severe reactions.
- Tick, and possibly mosquito, bites can produce infection with *Borrelia burgdorferi*, causing arthropathy, fever, and a distinctive rash (erythema chronicum migrans)—Lyme disease. The condition responds rapidly to treatment with penicillin. Increasing numbers of cases are being reported in the United Kingdom.

Papular urticaria

Persistent pruritic (itching) papules in groups on the trunk and legs may be due to bites from fleas, bed bugs, or mites.
A seasonal incidence suggests bites from outdoor insects, while recurrence of the papules in a particular house or room suggests infestations with fleas. The term is sometimes used for other causes of itchy skin.

Spider bites

In Europe spider bites rarely cause problems, but sometimes noxious species arrive in consignments of tropical fruit. The patient shown had been bitten by a spider the day before leaving Nigeria and developed a painful necrotic lesion.

Bites from the European tarantula are painful but otherwise harmless.

In tropical and subtropical countries venomous spiders inject neurotoxins that can be fatal. The "black widow" (*Latrodectus mactans*), "fiddleback" (*Loxosceles veclusa*), and *Atrax* species of Australia are better known examples. Scorpions cause severe local and systemic symptoms as a result of stings (not bites).

Infestations

Scabies

The commonest infestation encountered is scabies, and it is easily missed or misdiagnosed. Scabies is due to a small mite, *Sarcoptes scabiei*. The female mite burrows into the stratum corneum to lay

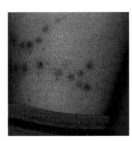

Bites on ankles

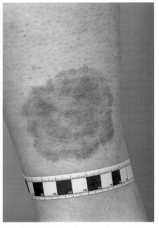

Erythema chronicum migrans

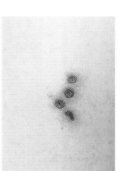

Harvest mites

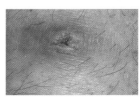

Spider bite (Nigeria)

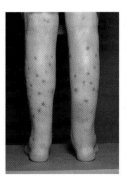

Papular urticaria

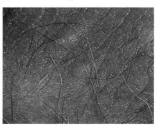

Persistent papules in scabies

her eggs; the male dies after completing his role of fertilisation, and the developing eggs hatch into larvae within a few days. Intense itching occurs some two weeks later, during which time extensive colonisation may have occurred. The infestation is acquired only by close contact with infected people.

Diagnosis

Finding a burrow—the small (5–10 mm long) ridge, often S shaped—can be difficult as it is often obscured by excoriation from scratching. Without finding a burrow, however, the diagnosis remains uncertain. Isolation of an acarus with a needle or scalpel blade and its demonstration under the microscope convinces the most sceptical patient. Always ask whether there are others in the patient's household and if any of them are itching.

Treatment

10% sulphur in yellow soft paraffin is traditional, effective, and safe. There are several more modern treatments, including 25% benzyl benzoate emulsion, 0·5% malathion cream, 1% gamma benzene hexachloride (lindane) lotion, and 1% permethrin. In children benzyl benzoate should be diluted to 10% and used with care as toxicity results from absorption. In infants over two months old permethrin or 2·5% sulphur ointment can be used. Gamma benzene hexachloride should not be given to children under 10 years or pregnant women in the first trimester. Important points are:

(1) The patient should wash well: a hot bath was formerly advocated but it is now known that this may increase absorption through the skin.
(2) The lotion should be applied from the neck down, concentrating on affected areas and making sure that the axillae, wrists, ankles, and pubic areas are included. If there is any doubt about the thoroughness of application the process should be repeated in a few days.
(3) All contacts and members of the patient's household should be treated at the same time.
(4) Residual papules may persist for many weeks. Topical steroids can be used to relieve the itching.
(5) Secondary infection as a result of scratching may need to be treated.

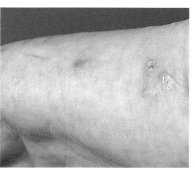

Burrows of scabies

> **Scabies—points to note**
> - There may be very few burrows, though the patient has widespread itching
> - The distribution of the infestation is characteristically the fingers, wrists, nipples, abdomen, genitalia, buttocks, and ankles
> - Close personal contact is required for infestation to occur, for example, within a family, through infants in playgroups, and through regular nursing of elderly patients
> - Itching may persist even after all mites have been eliminated; itching papules on the scrotum and penis are particularly persistent

Demodex

Demodex folliculorum is a small mite that inhabits the human hair follicle, the eggs being deposited in the sebaceous gland. It is found on the central area of the face, chest, and neck of adults. It may have a role in the pathogenesis of rosacea, in which it may be found in large numbers. It may be associated with a pustular eruption round the mouth and blepharitis.

Larva migrans

The patient in the illustration had been on holiday at a tropical coastal town and regularly visited a beach frequented by dogs. Two weeks after returning to Britain he started itching on the buttocks and subsequently noticed a linear, raised area—a condition known as larva migrans, due to the larvae of the hookworm of dogs and cats, *Ancylostoma caninum*. The ova are shed in the faeces and in a warm moist environment hatch into larvae that invade "dead end" hosts. They do not develop any further, so systemic disease does not occur.

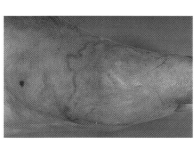

Larva migrans

Treatment

This is either by freezing the advancing end of the lesion with liquid nitrogen or by applying thiabendazole (10%) suspension. Similar lesions in patients returning from tropical countries raise the possibility of larva migrans from strongyloides infestation, myiasis from the larvae of flies, or gnathostomiasis.

Visceral larva migrans caused by *Toxocara canis* and *Ascaris lumbricoides* may produce a transient rash.

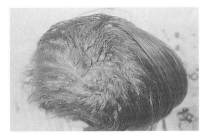
Pediculosis capitis

Pediculosts (lice)

Infestation with lice became less common in the postwar years, but the incidence has recently increased.

There are three areas of the body usually affected by two species of wingless insects—*Pediculus humanus,* infecting the head and body, and *Phthirus pubis,* the pubic louse. The wingless insects feed on blood aspirated at the site of the bite, and each female lays 60–80 encapsulated eggs attached to hairs—"nits" in common parlance.

Head lice are transmitted via combs, brushes, and hats, being more common in girls than boys. The infestation is heaviest behind the ears and over the occiput. If the eyelashes of children are affected this is with "crab lice" (*Phthlrus pubis*); it is not pediculosis.

Body lice are less common in western Europe. Transmission is by clothing and bedding, on which both lice and their eggs may be found in the seams. Poor hygiene favours infestation.

Pubic lice infestation occurs worldwide and is generally transmitted by sexual contact. Infestation of eyelashes may occur with poor hygiene.

As a result of scratching there may be marked secondary infection that obscures the underlying infestation.

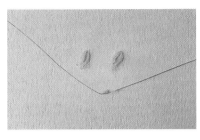
Head lice and nits

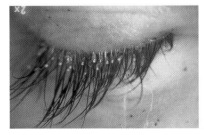
Phthirus pubis on eyelashes

Treatment

Gamma benzene hexachloride 1% is usually effective as a single application. Permethrin can also be used.

Further reading

Alexander JO. *Arthropods and human skin.* Berlin: Springer-Verlag, 1984

Busvine JR. *Insects and hygiene,* 3rd ed. London: Chapman and Hall, 1980

Marshall AG. *The ecology of ectoparasitic insects.* New York: Academic Press, 1981

Parish CL, Nutting WB, Schwartzman RM. *Cutaneous infestation of man and animal.* New York: Greenwood, 1983

23   Tropical dermatology

B Leppard

The purpose of this chapter is to provide an overview of tropical diseases that most commonly affect the skin. This will be useful for health workers who may not be familiar with tropical diseases and also as a guide to help those who are already working in the tropics and who see them all the time.

Skin disease is extemely common in the tropics, affecting up to 50% of the population. Most are infections or infestations such as impetigo, ringworm, and scabies. These can easily be treated but continue to be common because of overcrowding, poverty, and the lack of resources given to health care (training of health personnel and lack of basic medicines). To a large extent such diseases can be controlled with very simple measure suitable for use by those with minimal training. Atopic eczema is just as common in urban areas in the tropics as in the west. Skin cancers are uncommon in those with a black skin because of the protective effect of melanin, but are common in albinos.

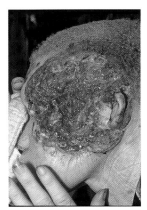
Albino with squamous cell carcinoma

The spectrum of tropical dermatology

All the common inflammatory dermatoses occur in the tropics but may have a different appearance in pigmented skin. Erythema, readily visible in Caucasians, will not be so apparent in black skin.

Infections and infestations occurring in the tropics produce distinctive skin changes These may be due to the presence of the organism, ova, or larvae in the skin. In other diseases a reaction to the organism produces a rash.

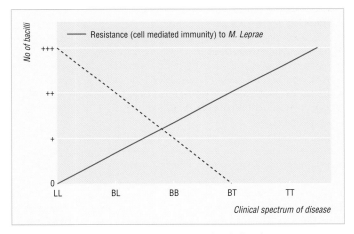

Spectrum of clinical disease in leprosy. (BB = borderline leprosy, BL = borderline lepromatous leprosy, BT = borderline tuberculoid leprosy, LL = lepromatous leprosy, TT = tuberculoid leprosy)

Bacterial infections

Impetigo is particularly prone to occur in the tropics and may complicate any area of minor trauma to the skin. It is characterised by erythema, and exudative lesions forming crusts.

Bullae may develop. If possible swabs should be taken for bacteriology and the appropriate antibiotics given.

Erysipelas is a localised streptococcal infection with erythema and tenderness accompanied by fever and malaise. Treatment is with penicillin.

Leprosy
Leprosy is a chronic infection of the skin and nerves by *Mycobacterium leprae*. It is spread by droplet infection and has a long incubation period (anything from two months to 40 years). There is a spectrum of clinical disease depending on the patient's cell mediated immunity to the organism.

Diagnosis
- *Typical clinical findings:*
  (a) In tuberculoid leprosy (TT) there is a single anaesthetic patch or plaque with a raised border.

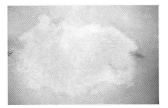
Tuberculoid leprosy

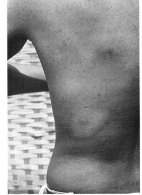
Tuberculoid leprosy

(b) In lepromatous leprosy (LL) there are widespread
symmetrical shiny papules, nodules, and plaques which
are not anaesthetic.

(c) In borderline leprosy (BT, BB, BL) there are varying
numbers of lesions, few in BT and numerous in BL.
They may be widespread but are asymmetrical.

(d) Palpably enlarged cutaneous nerves (great auricular
nerve in the neck, the superficial branch of the radial
nerve at the wrist, the ulnar nerve at the elbow, the
lateral popliteal nerve at the knee, and the sural nerve
on the lower leg).

(e) Glove and stocking sensory loss causing blisters, ulcers or
both on anaesthetic fingers or toes.

(f) Deformity due to invasion of the peripheral nerves with
leprosy bacilli, a leprosy reaction or recurrent trauma to
anaesthetic limbs.

- *Slit skin smears* measure the numbers of bacilli in the skin
(Bacterial Index (BI)) and the % of these that are living
(Morphological Index (MI)).

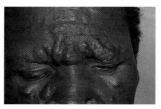
Lepromatous leprosy

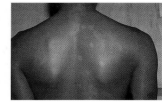
Borderline leprosy

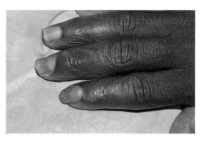
Borderline tuberculoid leprosy

Treatment
Paucibacillary leprosy (BI of 0 or 1+):
  Rifampicin 600 mg once a month (supervised) } for
  Dapsone 100 mg daily   } six months
Multibacillary leprosy (BI of 2+ or more):
  Rifampicin 600 mg once a month (supervised) ⎫
  Clofazamine 300 mg once a month   ⎪
    (supervised)   ⎬ for two years
  Clofazamine 50 mg/day   ⎪
  Dapsone 100 mg/day   ⎭

Cutaneous leishmaniasis

Cutaneous leishmaniasis is due to the protozoa *Leishmania
tropica*, and is transmitted by the bite of a sandfly. There is
a spectrum of disease depending on the patient's immunity.

Acute leishmaniasis
A red nodule like a boil occurs at the site of the bite.
It enlarges, may or may not ulcerate, and heals spontaneously
after about one year leaving a cribriform scar.

Chronic leishmaniasis
In a patient with good cell mediated immunity, after the acute
leishmaniasis has healed, new granulomata appear at the edge
of the scar; these do not heal spontaneously.

Diffuse cutaneous leishmaniasis
This is leishmaniasis in a patient with no immunity to the
organism (equivalent to lepromatous leprosy). Extensive skin
nodules occur that are full of organisms.

Treatment
Intramuscular injections of sodium stibogluconate 10 mg/kg
body weight daily until healing occurs.

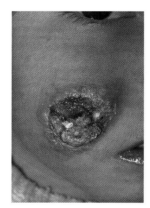
Acute leishmaniasis

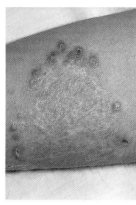
Chronic leishmaniasis

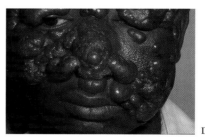
Diffuse cutaneous leishmaniasis

Superficial fungal infections

The same fungal infections of the epidermis occur in the tropics
as in temperate climates only more so—heat and occlusion of
clothing leading to maceration of the skin in which fungi thrive,
so expect to see more florid lesions. There are also many
fungal infections that are specifically found in the tropics.
These include tinea imbricata, tinea nigra, piedra, and
favus.

Bacterial Index (BI)

  0 = No bacilli seen
  1+ = 1–10 bacilli in 100 oil immersion fields
  2+ = 1–10 bacilli in 10 oil immersion fields
  3+ = 1–10 bacilli in 1 oil immersion field
  4+ = 10–100 bacilli in an average oil immersion field
  5+ = 100–1000 bacilli in an average oil immersion field
  6+ = >1000 bacilli in an average oil immersion field

Suspect a dermatophyte fungal infection in any chronic, itching, scaling, slowly developing lesion with epidermal changes.

Tinea imbricata due to *Tricophyton concentricum* is characterised by superficial concentric scaling rings spreading across the trunk. It occurs mainly in Asia but also in other tropical areas.

Tinea nigra occurs in the tropical areas of America, Asia, and Australia. Brown or black macules are seen on the palms and soles. It is due to *Cladosporium werneckii.*

Piedra is a fungal infection of the hair producing hard nodular lesions on the hair shaft. The lesions may be black (due to *Piedra hortai*) or white piedra (due to *Trichosporum beigelii*).

Favus is widespread throughout the Mediterranean, the Middle East, and tropics, but is rare in Africa. It is due to an endothrix fungus—*Trichophyton schoenleinii*—which causes a thick yellow crust with an unpleasant odour. Erythematous areas of scarring occur that must be differentiated from lichen planus and other causes of scarring alopecia.

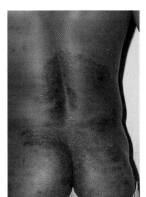
Superficial fungal infection

Deep fungal infections

In these conditions there is chronic inflammation in the subcutaneous tissues leading to granulomatous and necrotic nodules.

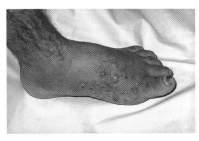
Tinea imbricata

Mycetoma (Madura foot)

This is a chronic infection of the dermis and subcutaneous fat caused by various species of fungus (*eumycetoma*) or bacteria (*actinomycetoma*). Both types look the same with a swollen foot and multiple discharging sinuses, but it is important to differentiate between them because the treatment is different.

Diagnosis
- Examination of the discharging grains (colour will give a clue as to the cause).
- Culture of the grains to identify the causative fungus or bacteria.
- If no grains can be found a skin biopsy will show them.

Treatment
Eumycetoma:

- Itraconazole 200 mg twice daily for at least 12 months if it is affordable.
  If not
- Surgical excision of affected tissue if disease is limited.
- Amputation if extensive.

Actinomycetoma:
- Sulfamethoxazole-trimethoprim mixture 960 mg twice daily for up to two years.

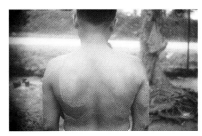
Madura foot

Blastomycosis

This condition is caused by the invasion of lymphatic system, lungs, and skin by *Paracoccioddes brasiliensis.* The widespread cutaneous lesions, which vary in appearance and distribution, must be differentiated from tuberculosis and other mycoses such as sporotrichosis, chromomycodis, and coccidiomycosis. It occurs in central and south America.

Chromomycosis
This chronic granulomatous condition mainly affects the legs and results from infestation by a variety of parasitic fungi. Large verrucous plaques may require surgical removal.

Histoplasmosis
This occurs in West Africa with nodules, ulcers, and bone lesions developing due to infection with *Histoplasma duboisii*. Treatment is with aphotericin B.

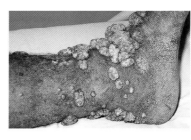

Chromomycosis

Infestations

Tungiasis
Invasion of the skin by sand fleas (*Tunga penetrans*) causes tungiasis in tropical areas of Africa, America, and India. It is most common on the feet, especially under the toes and toenails. The condition looks a bit like plantar warts, but if you watch for a while you will see the eggs being squirted out.

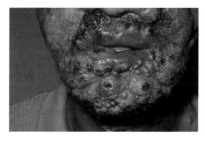

Histoplasmosis in HIV infection

Prevention
Wear shoes.

Treatment
- Carefully winkle the fleas out with a pin (most patients know how to do this themselves).
- If the fleas are very extensive, soak the feet in kerosene or treat with a single dose of ivermectin 200 micrograms/kg body weight.

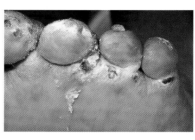

Tungiasis

Subcutaneous myiasis
Invasion of the skin by the larvae of the tumbu (mango) fly (*Cordylobia anthropophaga*) in central and southern Africa causes this condition. The fly lays her eggs on clothes layed out to dry on the ground. The eggs hatch out two days later on contact with the warm skin when the clothes are put on. The larvae burrow into the skin causing a red painful or itchy papule or nodule, predominantly on the trunk, buttocks, and thighs.

Other flies that cause miyasis are:

- *Dermatobia hominis*—tropical bot fly, in Mexico, central, and south America with tender nodules developing on the scalp, legs, forearms, and face.
- *Aucheronia* sp.—Congo floor maggot, in central and southern Africa. Bites of the larvae cause intense irritation.
- *Callitroga* sp. in central America causing inflamed lesions with necrosis.

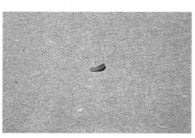

Myiasis—larvae

Prevention
Iron the clothes before wearing them.

Treatment
Cover the nodule with petroleum jelly or other grease; the larva will be unable to breath and will crawl out.

Filariasis
This is an infestation with thread-like helminths (Latin "Filum"—a thread). They are widely distributed in many species and live in the lymphatics and connective tissue. Fertilised eggs develop into embryonic worms—microfilariae. These are taken up by insect vectors that act as intermediate hosts in which further development occurs. They are then inoculated into a human host when next bitten by the insect.

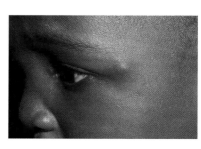

Myiasis—papule

Three diseases are caused by filarial worms:

- Lymphatic filariasis due to *Wuchereria bancrofti*, which liberate microfilariae into the blood stream.
- Onchocerciasis due to *Onchocera volvulus*. The microfilariae are liberated into the skin and subcutaneous tissues.
- Loiasis due to *Loa loa*, in which microfilariae are found in the blood.

Lymphatic filariasis affects 120 million people in 73 countries (34% in sub-Saharan Africa). It causes lymphoedema of the legs, genitalia, and breasts. It may be asymptomatic for a long period and the adult worms live for four to six years in the lymphatic vessels and lymph nodes producing thousands of microfilaria each day. These are picked up by mosquitoes when they take a blood meal and are passed on to the next victim when they feed again.

Treatment
- In endemic areas the whole community should be treated with a single dose of two of the following three drugs once a year for four to six years:
  (a) Ivermectin 400 micrograms/kg body weight
  (b) Diethylcarbamazine (DEC) 6 mg/kg body weight
  (c) Albendazole 600 mg.
- The chronic lymphoedema can be improved by keeping the legs moving, raising the legs when sitting, and prevention of secondary bacterial infection by regular washing and moisturising of the skin.

Onchocerciasis
Onchocerciasis (river blindness) occurs in Africa south of the Sahara and in Central America. It is due to *Onchocerca volvulus* transmitted by the bite of black flies Simuliidae which breed by fast flowing rivers. The inoculation of microfilariae by the bite of a black fly causes intense local inflammation and is followed by an incubation period of many months. The adult worms live in nodules around the hips and cause no harm in themselves. They produce thousands of microfilaria each day which travel to the skin and eyes. In the skin they produce a very itchy rash which looks like lichenified eczema. On the lower legs there is often spotty depigmentation. Involvement of the eyes causes blindness.

Risk factors for being infected
- Living, working, or playing near fast flowing rivers.
- Not wearing enough clothes so that the skin is exposed to insect bites.
- The construction of dams leads to less breeding of black flies in the dam itself but increased breeding in the dam spillways.

Diagnosis
- Demonstrate the microfilaria in the skin by skin snips.
- Remove a skin nodule and see the adult worms inside it.
- Polymerase chain reaction to show parasite DNA—not much use in the field.

Treatment

- Spray the breeding areas with insecticides.
- Annual dose of ivermectin 400 micrograms/kg body weight for four to six years. This stops the release of microfilaria from the adult worms.

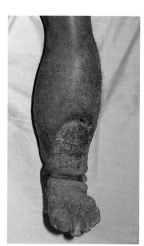
Lymphoema of the legs in filariasis

Diagnosis
- Find the microfilaria on a thick blood smear taken at midnight. This is not a very convenient method of diagnosis.
- Immuno-chromatographic filariasis card test using finger prick blood, which takes less than five minutes to complete. It detects circulating *W. bancrofti* antigens so it can be done at any time of the day or night.
- Polymerase chain reaction to detect parasitic DNA. This is very sensitive and can detect as little as one microfilaria in 1 ml blood.

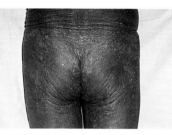
Onchocerciasis

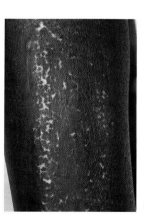
"Leopard skin" in onchocerciasis

Loiasis

Loiasis occurs in the rain forests of central and west Africa. It is transmitted by mango flies (*Chrysops*). The adult worms live in the subcutaneous tissues where they can be seen in the skin and under the conjunctiva. The microfilaria are only found in the blood. A hypersensitivity to the worms shows itself as swelling of the skin, particularly of the wrists and ankles (calabar swellings).

Dracontiasis

This condition is due to infestation by *Draculus medinensis* in the connective tissue. It is acquired from drinking water containing the intermediate host, a crustacean, *Cyclops*. Localised papules develop on the lower legs containing the female worm and numerous microfilariae. Treatment consists of very carefully extracting the worm by winding it onto a stick over several weeks. Symptomatic treatment of secondary infection and allergic reactions is also required.

Diagnosis of loiasis

- Find the microfilaria in the peripheral blood between 10 am and 2 pm
- Find the adult worms by ultrasound examination
- High blood eosinophilia

Treatment of loiasis

- A single dose of ivermectin 400 micrograms/kg body weight or a three week course of albendazole 400 mg/kg body weight/bd
- Do not use diethylcarbamazine citrate (DEC) as this can cause death as a result of a reaction to toxins from the rapid destruction of the microfilaria.

24 Practical procedures and where to use them

DWS Harris

Skin lesions are easily accessible for removal or biopsy. The procedure used needs to be appropriate to the site and type of lesion involved. It is important also to keep scarring to a minimum.

Destruction of skin lesions is carried out with:
- Electrocautery
- Cryotherapy
- Laser treatment

This is suitable for lesions where the diagnosis is certain, as no specimen is available or histology.

Removal of skin lesions results in a specimen for the pathologist to examine. The techniques used are:

- Curettage and cautery
- Surgical excision
- Incisional biopsy which provides a specimen for histology to supplement the clinical diagnosis.

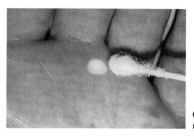

Cryotherapy—applying the liquid nitrogen

Cryotherapy

This involves the destruction of tissues by extreme cold. Current methods used are:

Carbon dioxide
Solid carbon dioxide (temperature $-64\,°C$) is produced by allowing rapid expansion of the compressed gas from a cylinder. This can be mixed with acetone to form a slush that can be applied with a cotton wool bud. A solid carbon dioxide stick, for direct application to lesions, is produced by an apparatus using "sparklet" bulbs.

The lesion must be frozen solid with a 1–2 mm margin of surrounding tissue. After thawing the freezing cycle should be repeated.

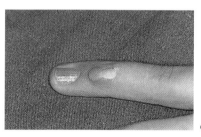

Cryotherapy—the frozen wart

Liquid nitrogen ($-196\,°C$)
This can be simply applied using a cotton wool bud dipped in the vacuum flask of liquid nitrogen. Freezing takes a little longer than using spray apparatus. Various types of such apparatus are available with different sizes of nozzle. The larger ones are used for seborrhoeic keratoses on the back, for example, and the smaller sizes for small lesions on the face. Freezing takes a few seconds and after thawing a further application can be made if necessary.

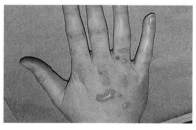

Cryotherapy—subsequent slight blistering

Ethyl chloride
This is sprayed directly on the skin, producing lowering of the temperature and temporary analgesia. It is not generally used for treatment.

Nitrous oxide
A cylinder of compressed gas is used to cool a probe to approximately $-80\,°C$. It is usually used for the treatment of warts and requires a 30 second freezing cycle.

Precautions
- Cryotherapy produces pain and inflammation. Blistering and haematoma may occur. This can be diminished by the

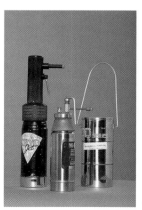

Cryotherapy—liquid nitrogen containers

application of a strong steroid cream immediately after freezing, except when treating viral warts as it tends to encourage proliferation of the warts.

- Damage to deeper structures is rare but may occur when freezing the deeper tissues—for example, treating basal cell carcinoma.
- It is possible for adjacent structures to be damaged accidentally, especially with the liquid nitrogen spray. This applies particularly when treating lesions on the face, when it is essential to screen the eyes adequately.

Skin lesions suitable for freezing

Viral warts
These may require several treatments at two to three week intervals. Freezing very small plane warts can result in small depigmented areas, so they may be better treated with wart paint.

Seborrhoeic keratoses
These respond well to cryotherapy, but as they are superficial lesions care must be taken to avoid excessive freezing with resultant scars.

Papillomata and skin tags
These can be easily and permanently treated by compression with artery forceps dipped in liquid nitrogen. Surprisingly, this is generally a painless procedure.

Dysplastic lesions
Early lesions, which are potentially neoplastic or of low grade malignancy, can be effectively treated. This includes solar keratoses, if early and superficial, but follow up is essential. The lesions can progress to squamous carcinoma, and if not responding to cryotherapy they should be excised or removed with curettage and cautery for histological examination.

Bowen's disease
An intraepidermal carcinoma, if confirmed by incisional biopsy, can respond to repeated cryotherapy. Follow up is essential since progression to an invasive squamous carcinoma can occur.

Basal cell carcinoma
The superficial spreading type can be treated with liquid nitrogen, but repeated and often prolonged freezing is required. To be certain of effective treatment a thermocouple probe to record the temperature at the base of the tumour is used. This is not usually a routine procedure in general practice or hospital outpatients. Excision or radiotherapy are more effective methods of treatment.

Electrocautery

There are two forms of treatment:

(1) Heat from an electrically heated element, which is used for removal of skin tags and for treatment of the surface after curettage of warts, also seborrhoeic keratoses.
(2) High energy, low current "electrodesiccation" equipment which produces a high energy spark that can coagulate blood vessels or destroy some more papillomata. A fine needle point should be used for small telangiectatic naevi or milia. A larger needle is used for larger surfaces, for example after curettage.

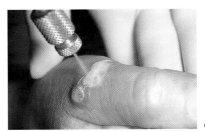

Cryotherapy—practical points
- Be sure of the diagnosis before cryotherapy, taking a biosy if necessary
- Explain to the patient that inflammation, blistering, or haematoma formation may occur
- Use freezing with care in children and on areas where the skin is thin, such as below the eyelids. In pigmented skin postinflammatory hyperpigmentation can occur

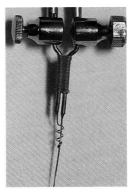

Cryotherapy—freezing a lesion

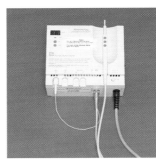

Electrocautery—pinpoint cautery attachment

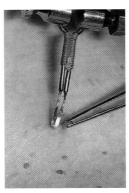

Electrocautery—pinpoint cautery attachment

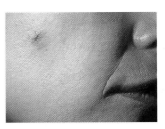

Electrocautery—hyfrecator

Electrocautery—spider naevus

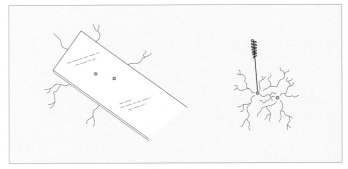

Electrocautery—blanch the lesion to identify feeding vessels, then insert the needle into feeding vessels in the cold state

Laser treatment

Laser—Light Amplification by Stimulated Emission of Radiation—produces high energy radiation. The first laser apparatus was developed from microwave technology in 1960 by the nobel prize winner TH Mamian. It was initially used as a destructive tool to ablate tumours, but now different wavelengths can be directed at specific targets. Blood vessels, for example, take up the blue/green light of the argon laser and the red light of a ruby laser is well absorbed by the green dye of tattoos. Modern developments have resulted in laser equipment that produces minimal scarring and maximum specificity.

Although smaller portable units are available, laser treatment should still only be undertaken by those with appropriate training. The skin lesions most commonly treated by laser are described below.

Tattoos

Tattoos contain a variety of pigments so that more than one type of laser may be necessary for complete removal. The same pigment may vary in response in different patients. Superficial dark pigment usually responds to the Q switch ruby laser, but deeper pigment may require the Nd:YAG laser or Alexandrite laser. Green pigment is usually removed with a Q switch ruby laser and red pigment with a green light laser such as the Q switched Nd:YAG. It is found that professional tattoos are usually more easily removed than the amateur type.

Pigmented lesions

Melanin absorbs light over a wide range of wavelengths, which can result in undesirable loss of skin colour following laser treatment. This can be put to good use in the treatment of benign lentigines and café au lait patches or deeply seated pigmented naevi. A wide range of laser types can be used, including Q switch ruby and Nd:YAG lasers. Congenital pigmented naevi should not be treated unless the biopsy has confirmed that they are benign.

Hair follicles

Laser equipment is available for removing excess hair and is a very effective cosmetic tool.

Laser surgery

Lasers can be used as a cutting tool and recent studies have shown them to be a very effective means of producing incisions in the skin.

Curettage

This is a simple way of removing epidermal lesions. A curette has a metal spoon shaped end with a sharp cutting edge. There are a variety of shapes and sizes suitable for different lesions, from large seborrhoeic keratoses or papillomata to smaller ones for minute keratin cysts. A specimen is provided for histology but completeness of removal cannot be accurately assessed.

Treatment of vascular lesions

- **Port wine stains**
  Argon and carbon dioxide lasers cause scarring, so yellow light emitting types such as Krypton, Flashlamp Powered Dye Laser (FIPDL), or Copper Laser are used
- **Telangiectasia**
  This is also treated with the FIPDL, although this can cause transient purpura, or Copper Laser
- **Cavernous haemangioma**
  These can be treated by yellow dye laser followed by surgical excision

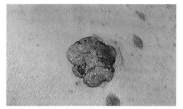

Curettage—seborrhoeic keratosis

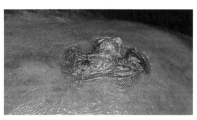

Curettage—actinic keratosis

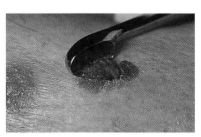

Curettage

Lesions suitable for curetting

- Seborrhoeic keratoses
- Solitary viral warts
- Solar keratoses
- Cutaneous horns
- Small basal cell carcinomas

Local anaesthetic is used and, with the skin stretched, the curette is applied at the edge of the lesion which is then scooped off. It is advisable to work around the edges of larger or more firmly attached lesions. The dermis normally feels firm but when curetting off a keratotic horn or solar keratoses; a soft consistency may indicate dysplastic change. The base can be lightly cauterised to control bleeding, sterilise the site, and prevent recurrence.

Various types of disposable curettes are available and are easy to use.

Curettage and cautery

- Use a sharp curette of appropriate size
- Very firm control of the curette prevents it from suddenly skidding onto normal skin
- Repeat curettage and cautery for neoplastic lesions such as basal cell carcinoma and solar keratoses
- Send the specimen for pathological examination

Incisional biopsy and punch biopsy

It is essential to have a working clinical diagnosis, but wherever there is doubt the pathologists can provide much more precise information regarding the nature and extent of the lesion. For example, a patch of Bowen's disease (intraepidermal carcinoma) may resemble sclerosing superficial basal cell carcinoma and a biopsy will usually distinguish them. Similarly, what seems to be a dysplastic pigmented naevus clinically may, on the one hand, prove to be benign or, on the other hand, turn out to be a malignant melanoma requiring wide excision.

Immunofluorescent staining of a blistering lesion differentiates dermatitis herpetiformis, which is treated with a gluten free diet, from pemphigoid, which requires corticosteroids and often immunosuppressant drugs.

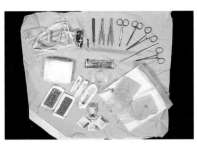

Biopsy—equipment needed

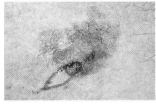

Incisional biopsy—marking lesion

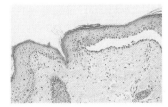

Incisional biopsy—histology

Incisional biopsy
This is suitable for larger lesions and is taken across the margin of the lesion in the form of an elipse. It is essential to include deeper dermis, as the significant changes in, for example, granuloma or lymphoid infiltrate may not be near the surface. An adequate amount of normal tissue should be included, so this could be compared with the pathological area and this also means there is enough normal skin to suture the incision together.

Punch biopsy
The biopsy tool consists of a small cylinder with a cutting rim which is used to penetrate the epidermis by rotation between the operator's finger and thumb. There is minimal danger of damaging deeper structures as the elastic subcutaneous tissues merely rotate with the tool without being cut. The resulting plug of skin is lifted out with forceps and cut off as deeply as possible.

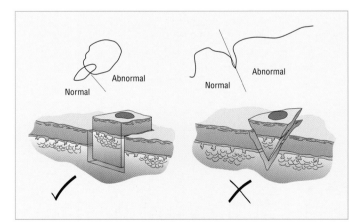

Incisional biopsy—amount of tissue that should be taken

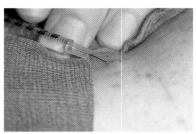

Punch biopsy—injecting local anaesthetic

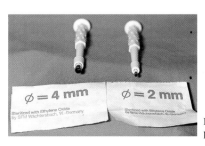

Punch biopsy—examples of punches

With the smaller sized punches the resulting defect can be treated with electrocautery or left to heal spontaneously. With a punch larger than 3 or 4 mm a single suture can be used. The main disadvantage of a punch biopsy is that it only provides a single small piece of tissue. It may not be representative or may miss an area of substantial change. It tends to leave a more prominent scar than the incisional biopsy.

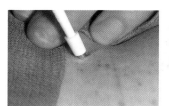

Punch biopsy—tool inserted

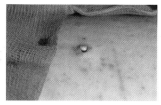

Punch biopsy—plug of skin

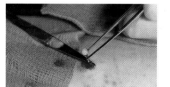

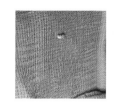

Punch biopsy—raising plug of skin to cut

Punch biopsy—treating defect with electrocautery

Punch biopsy—specimen taken

Excision of skin lesions is both curative and diagnostic. It may be the best way of making a diagnosis if there are multiple small papules or vesicles, one of which can be excised intact. Incisions should follow tension or wrinkle lines.

In the case of malignant lesions it is particularly important that the whole lesion is adequately excised. The pathologist can report on the adequacy of excision, but not in multifocal basal cell carcinoma where this cannot be assessed. If there is likely to be any doubt about the excision being complete it is helpful to attach a suture to one end of the excised specimen so the pathologist can describe which border, if any, extends over the excision margin.

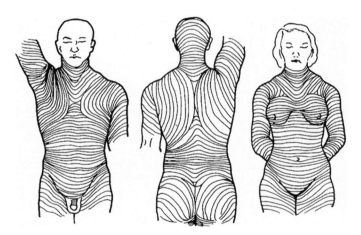

Surgical excision—"wrinkle lines" of skin

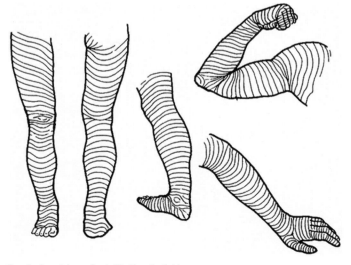

Surgical excision—"wrinkle lines" of skin

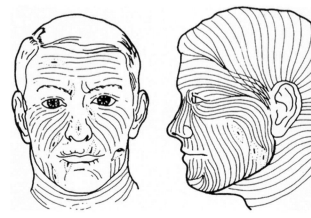

Surgical excision—"wrinkle lines" of skin

Technique

The basic technique consists of making an elliptical incision
with the length three times the width. This enables suturing
without the formation of "dog ears" at the end. The long axis
of the excision should follow the "wrinkle lines" of the skin,
which are parallel to the collagen bundle in the dermis. This
produces stronger, narrower scars. They are not the same as the
deeper lines or fasical attachment or "Lange lines". Lesions on
the sternal area, upper chest, and shoulders, where keloid scars
often form, should only be excised when it is essential and may
be best referred to a plastic surgeon.

Local anaesthetic is injected subcutaneously but close to the
skin. The incision should be vertical rather than wedge shaped.
Monofilament sutures cause less inflammation and trapping of
serum than the braided variety, but are harder to tie securely.

Methods of suturing and the more specialised techniques of
flaps and grafts are outside the scope of this book. It is an asset
for the dermatologist to be able to carry out surgical procedures
on the skin and suitable courses are generally available.

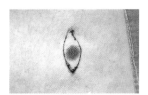
Surgical excision—elliptical
incision

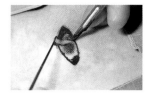
Surgical excision—raising skin

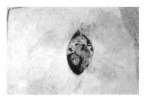
Surgical excision—appearance
of lesions under skin

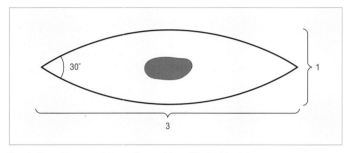
Surgical excision—guidance for making elliptical incision

Surgical excision

- After initially inserting the needle, withdraw the plunger of
  the syringe to check the needle has not entered the blood
  vessels. Raising a small "bleb" of local anaesthetic ahead of
  the needle point helps to prevent this
- It is important to learn appropriate suturing techniques for
  different sites of the body and size of lesion
- Warn the patient that a scar will result and make sure that
  this is minimal and does not produce any deformity such as
  displacement of the eyelid
- Always send an excised lesion for histology. A significant
  number of lesions diagnosed as being benign clinically have
  been shown to be malignant. This would of course be missed
  if they had not been sent to a laboratory

Further reading

Lawrence C. *Introduction to dermatological surgery.* Oxford: Blackwell
Science, 1997

Tromovitch TA, Stegman SJ, Glogau RG. *Flaps and grafts in
dermatologic surgery.* Chicago: Year Book Medical, 1989

Zachary CB. *Basic cutaneous surgery: a primer in technique.* New York:
Churchill Livingstone, 1991

25 Dermatology in general practice

R Balfour, E Crawford

In common with other aspects of general practice the management of dermatological problems has changed considerably in recent years. In particular:

- There is an increased expectation from patients, who want an accurate diagnosis and prompt treatment but also expect treatment for even the smallest lesion.
- The management of inflammatory skin conditions no longer requires many weeks of inpatient treatment. "Daily dressing clinics" in hospital dermatology departments enable patients to continue their daily lives while being treated, but still require visits to hospital. In many practices facilities for carrying out dressings by the practice nurse have been developed.
- The demand for specialist services far outstrips supply. Consequently the majority of patients with skin conditions have to be treated by general practitioners. One positive outcome is that there is a greater emphasis on shared care between general practice and hospital specialist departments. This is facilitated by the appointment of dermatology liaison nurses who are able to supervise patient's treatment in the community and, as the name suggests, liaise with both general practice and hospital departments using the resources of each as appropriate.
- General practitioners are increasingly developing special interests and many have part-time posts in specialist departments. In the case of dermatology this enhances their clinical knowledge, which they can bring to bear on the problems in general practice.

Between 10% and 15% of consultations in general practice are for skin related problems, although the actual number of skin conditions seen is probably much higher than this. In one general practice an analysis of 100 consecutive consultations showed that 38 involved some aspect of dermatology. Increasing knowledge of dermatology enables conditions to be diagnosed and treated. Even if the diagnosis is not known it is important to be able to assess the probable importance of dermatological conditions and differentiate those for whom an urgent referral to hospital is required from those needing a specialist opinion to confirm the diagnosis and treatment but for whom there is no great urgency. This is important with the large demands being made on hospital departments with diminished funding and increasing waiting times. In this respect a good working relationship with the local hospital department is a great asset.

Diagnosis of skin conditions in general practice

As in all aspects of medicine, knowing how the more common conditions present will provide a basis for recognising the unusual variants or less common lesions. Psoriasis, eczema, and other forms of dermatitis usually present no problems. Where they do a review of the history often gives valuable clues. Atopic eczema in childhood may explain the development of a widespread itching rash in a young adult and an otherwise unexplained rash may well be accounted for after a review of

Dermatology in general practice

- In a study of one area of London 55% of adults examined had some form of skin disease*
- Of those with moderate or severe conditions only 24% had made use of medical facilities in the previous six months
- In the same study 30% of patients with skin conditions medicated themselves
- Eight per cent of patients attending a general practitioner for a skin condition are referred to a dermatologist†
- A large reservoir of people in the community with skin conditions do not seek medical attention but can be expected to do so as awareness of skin conditions increases‡
- General practitioners with postgraduate training in dermatology and dermatology liaison nurses linked to specialist centres are needed so that the increasing demand for dermatology services can be met
- In countries with specialist care, basic training in the essentials of daignosis and treatment of skin conditions enables health officers to make a considerable impact on these conditions in the community

*Rea JN, Newhouse ML, Halil T. Skin disease in Lambeth: a community study of prevalence and use of medical care. *Br J Prev Soc Med* 1976;30:107-14
†Carmichael AJ. Achieving an accessible dermatology service. *Dermatol Pract* 1995;3:13-16
‡Savin J. The hidden face of dermatology. *Clin Exp Dermatol* 1999;18:393-5

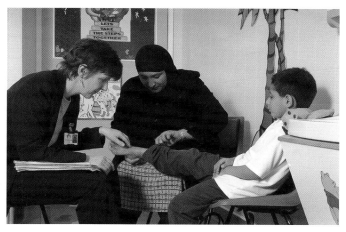

Hospital consultation

current drugs the patient is taking. Knowledge of the dermatological conditions associated with systemic disease, and conditions that may mimic them, is clearly important. A bilateral malar rash with photosensitivity in a woman should suggest the possibility of lupus erythematosus and appropriate investigations instituted. However, a completely typical case of rosacea does not require extensive investigation. The most useful diagnostic aids in general practice are:

- Skin scrapings and a sellotape strip should be sent for mycology whenever there is an area of itching inflammatory change, particularly in the flexures, that is not responding to treatment.
- A swab for bacteriology should be sent from any area of dermatitis that develops crusting and exudate.
- An incisional biopsy can be carried out to confirm a significant diagnosis, for example in a patch of Bowen's disease This is not usually needed to make a diagnosis of granuloma annulare, which has a very characteristic presentation. All lesions removed by excision or curettage or cautery should be sent for histology.
- Patch testing is not practicable in general practice as a rule because of the large number of reagents and specialised nursing skills required. Patients suspected of having contact dermatitis should be referred to the appropriate unit.

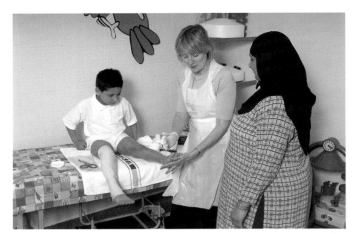

Demonstration of dressings by liaison nurse

The management of skin conditions in general practice

One great advantage of general practice is that there is continuity of care and the family doctor has a much more complete overall picture of the patient, their family and social circumstances than can be acquired in a hospital consultation. Increasingly dressings and other treatments are being used by practice nurses in conjunction with the dermatology liaison nurse when necessary. This applies to inflammatory skin conditions such as psoriasis and eczema as well as leg ulcers, but also to conditions such as Darier's disease, dermatitis herpetiformis, and lupus erythematosus where regular supervision and blood tests may be required. There is no reason why continuing treatment with drugs such as ciclosporin and methotrexate cannot be carried out in general practice once the diagnosis and treatment regime have been established. Regular blood tests are mandatory when these drugs are being used.

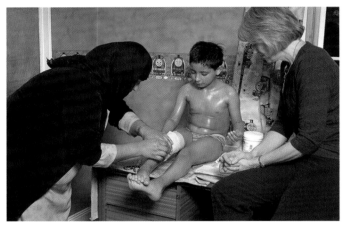

Dressings being applied at home by mother

Procedures in general practice

The details of techniques decribed in chapter 24.

- *Excisions* and other forms of minor surgery are probably best undertaken by a member of the practice who has developed expertise in this area, and received some level of training. It is particularly important to be aware of which lesions and anatomical sites are the most difficult for minor surgery. It is probably wise not to attempt excisions over the sternum and shoulders, particularly in young people, where keloid scars will probably result. In general it is best to refer any malignant lesion to a hospital department for excision.
- *Curettage and cautery* is a straightforward procedure for the removal of superficial and well defined lesions such as seborrhoeic keratoses and viral warts. It is as well to send all specimens for histology—to confirm the diagnosis and make sure that an unsuspected malignancy is not missed. It is important that a clinical probable diagnosis is made so as to

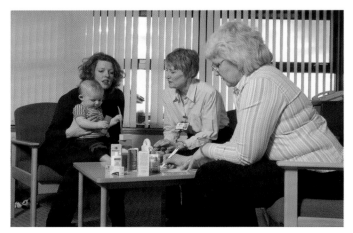

Mother, liaison nurse, and health visitor discuss treatment

avoid excising lesions where such treatment is not required or when it is inappropriate.

- *Cryotherapy* is suitable for the treatment of warts, seborrheoic keratoses, solar keratoses, and conditions such as Bowen's disease. If there is doubt as to the diagnosis or the condition fails to respond to treatment a specialist opinion should be sought. It usually most satisfactory to have a cryotherapy clinic for which liquid nitrogen is regularly supplied and a suitably trained nurse is available to carry out the treatment. It is important that all patients are seen by by a doctor before treatment is started so that the diagnosis and suitability for treatment can be confirmed.

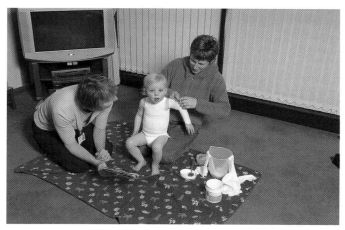

Mother applying wet wraps at home

Self-help groups

There are now groups that provide an invaluable source of information and advice for a wide range of conditions. A number of these are listed in the appendix.

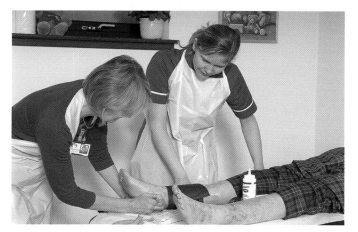

Assessment of circulation in leg ulcers by liaison nurse

Further reading

Barker DJ, Millard LG. *Essentials of skin disease management.* Oxford: Blackwell Scientific, 1979

Lamberg SI. *Dermatology in primary care: a problem oriented guide.* Philadelphia: Saunders, 1986

Stone LA, Lindfield EM, Robertson SJ. *A colour atlas of nursing procedures in skin disorders.* London and St. Louis: Mosby–Wolfe, 1989

26 Formulary

The zinc topped tables used for many years to prepare tar "spreads" in a teaching hospital dermatology department were recently thrown out—a sign of the times and an indication of both the increasing use of systemic treatment and much more effective forms of phototherapy. There is still an important place for topical treatment and "dressing clinics" to play a vital role in the treatment of skin diseases and enabling affected individuals to continue their daily lives as far as possible.

The link between hospital departments and community services has been greatly increased by the development of the role of "liaison nurses". These nurses, with experience and training in the treatment of skin disease, visit patients in their homes to supervise treatment in conjuction with the general practitioner and the practice nurse. As they are based in the hospital they can call on any specialist opinion or treatment needed.

A great variety of preparations is available for the treatment of skin conditions, and those most commonly used are described. There are numerous effective alternatives.

The techniques for the treatment of specific conditions are described in the appropriate chapters.

Topical treatment

General treatments
The epidermis is capable of absorbing both greasy and aqueous preparations or a mixture of the two. The type of lesion influences which type is used.

- Dry, scaling skin—greasy ointments.
- Crusted, weeping lesions—creams which are an emulsion of greases in water.
- For occlusion or long action—pastes which are powder (for example, zinc oxide) in an ointment.
- For the face and scalp—gels

Composition of bases
The consistency and properties of ointment and cream depend on the ratio of oil or grease to water (that is, whether they are oil in water or water in oil) and the emulsifying agents used. For example, emulsifying ointment contains soft white paraffin, emulsifying ointment, and liquid paraffin.

The oils and greases range from mineral oil through soft paraffin to solid waxes. Some are naturally occurring, such as lanolin and beeswax. Creams or ointments may be used on their own as emollients or as vehicles for active ingredients.

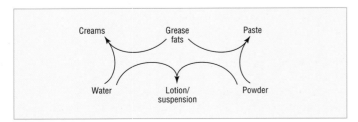

Composition of bases

Emollients
There are numerous preparations for softening dry scaling skin and it is largely a matter of personal preference as to which one is used.

Official preparations
- Soft white paraffin—greasy; protects skin and is long lasting.
- Emulsifying ointment—less greasy; mixes with water and can be used for washing.
- Aqueous cream—oil in water emulsion; useful as a vehicle, as an emollient, and for washing.
- Liquid paraffin: white soft paraffin, equal parts—spreads easily and is less greasy than white soft paraffin.
- Hydrophilic ointment—contains propylene glycol; mixes with water and spreads easily.
- Lanolin (hydrous wool fat)—the natural emollient from sheep; mixes with water and greases, softens the epidermis, but can also cause allergic reactions.

Proprietary preparations
Proprietary preparations are numerous, varied, and more expensive than the standard preparations. They may also contain sensitisers—lanolin and preservatives (hydroxybenzoate, chlorocresol, sorbic acid)—and can cause allergies. Some examples are E45 cream (Crookes), Oilatum cream (Stiefel), and Lacticare (Stiefel), Unguentum Merck (Merck), Aquadrate (Norwich Eaton), and Diprobase (Schering-Plough).

Bath additives
Bath additives comprise dispersible oils such as Oilatum (Westwood, United States), Aveeno (Bioglan), Balneum (Merck), Alpha Keri (Westwood, United States), Emulsiderm, and Dermol (Dermal).

Topical steroids
Topical steroids provide effective anti-inflammatory treatment but have the disadvantage of causing atrophy (due to decreased fibrin formation) and telangiectasis. They are readily absorbed by thin skin around the eyes and in flexures. On the face the halogenated steroids produce considerable telangiectasia, so nothing stronger than hydrocortisone should be used (except in lupus erythematosus). They can cause hirsutism and folliculitis or acne. Infection of the skin may be concealed (tinea incognita, for example) or made worse.

Side effects can be avoided by observing the following guidelines:

- Avoid long term use of strong steroids.
- Potent or very potent steroids should be applied sparingly and often for a short time, then a less potent preparation less often as the condition improves.
- Use only mildly potent steroids (that is, hydrocortisone) on the face.
- Use preparations combined with antibiotics or antifungals for the flexures.

Topical steroids come in various strengths and a wide variety of bases—ointments, creams, oily creams, lotions, and gels—which can be used according to the type of lesion being treated.

Their pharmacological activity varies and they are classified according to their potency, the synthetic halogenated steroids being much stronger than hydrocortisone:

- Mildly potent—hydrocortisone 0·5%, 1%, and 2·5%
- Moderately potent—Eumovate (GSK), Stiedex LP (Stiefel)
- Potent—Betnovate (GSK), Cutivate (GSK), Locoid (Brocades), Synalar (Zeneca)
- Very potent—Dermovate (GSK).

In Britain a full list showing relative potencies appears in MIMS. Combinations with antiseptics and antifungals, are listed below:

Mildly potent
- Vioform HC (Zyma)
- Terra-Cortril ointment (Pfizer), containing oxytetracycline and hydrocortisone
- Fucidin H cream or ointment (Leo), containing fucidic acid and hydrocortisone
- Canesten HC (Baypharm)
- Daktacort cream (Janssen)

Moderately potent
- Betnovate N (betamethasone and neomycin) (GSK)
- Synalar N (neomycin; Zeneca)
- Trimovate cream (clobetasone butyrate, nystatin, and oxytetracyclin; GSK)
- Fucibet (betamethasone, fucidic acid; Leo)

Very potent
- Dermovate-NN (clobetasone, with neomycin and nystatin; GSK).

Antiseptics and cleaning lotions

Simple antiseptics are very useful for cleaning infected, weeping lesions and leg ulcers.

Potassium permanganate can be used by dropping four or five crystals in a litre of water or in an 0·1% solution that is diluted to 0·01% for use as a soak. It will stain the skin temporarily and plastic containers permanently.

Silver nitrate 0·25% is a simple, safe antiseptic solution that, applied as a wet compress, is useful for cleaning ulcers.

Flamazine (Smith and Nephew) is silver sulfadiazine cream, used for leg ulcers, pressure sores, and burns.

Hydrogen peroxide (6%) helps remove slough but tends to be painful. Hioxyl (Quinoderm) is a proprietary cream for desloughing.

Iodine (2·5%) is an old fashioned, effective preparation as a tincture in alcohol and Betadine (Napp) is a proprietary equivalent.

Shampoos. Ceanel concentrate (Quinoderm) contains cetrimide 10%. Ionil T (Galderma) has benzalkonium chloride and coal tar solution, and Betadine (SSL) contains povidone iodine. Shampoos containing selenium sulphide (Selsun, Abbot) and ketokonazole (Nizoral, Janssen) can be used for seborrhoeic dermatitis and also for pityriasis versicolor of the skin.

There are numerous other antiseptic, cleansing, and desloughing agents such as cetrimide, chlorhexidine, benzalkonium chloride, benzoic acid, and enzyme preparations such as Varidase (Lederle), a streptokinase and streptodornase preparation.

Tar preparations

These are mainly used for treating psoriasis as described in chapter 3.

Tar has an anti-inflammatory effect and seems to suppress the epidermal turnover in lesions of psoriasis. The various tar pastes are generally too messy to use at home and are most suitable for dermatology treatment centres. Standard tar paste contains a strong solution of coal tar 7·5% in 25 g of zinc oxide, 25 g of starch, and 50 g of white soft paraffin.

There are numerous proprietary preparations that are less messy and do not stain but are not so effective. They are useful for treating less severe psoriasis at home. Examples are: Alphosyl cream (Stafford-Miller), Pragmatar (Bioglan), Psoriderm (Dermal); alphosyl HC (Stafford-Miller) and Carbo-Cort (Lagap) contain hydrocortisone as well.

Dithranol can be used in a paste containing salicylic acid, zinc oxide starch, and soft white paraffin. It has to be applied carefully avoiding contact with the surrounding skin, as it can cause severe irritation. It is best to start with a low concentration.

For short contact treatment relatively clean preparations in a range of concentrations are available, such as Dithrocream (Dermal), Anthranol (Stiefel), and Psoradrate cream (Stafford-Miller).

Ichthammol is a useful soothing extract of shale tar. It can be made up as a 1% paste in yellow soft paraffin with 15% zinc oxide.

Bath preparations are useful for dry skin and widespread psoriasis. Coal tar solution (20%) can be used or Polytar Emollient (Stiefel) or Psoriderm.

Tar shampoos are useful for treating psoriasis of the scalp. Polytar (Stiefel), T-Gel (Neutrogena), Capasal (Dermal), and Alphosyl (Stafford-Miller) are some examples.

Keratolytics

These can be used for hyperkeratotic lesions. They soften and help remove excess keratin. If used for extensive areas or in infants systemic absorption can occur. A useful preparation is salicylic acid 2–4% in aqueous cream. Salicylic acid with betamethasone ointment (Diprosalic ointment, Schering-Plough) can be used for hyperkeratotic lesions where inflammation is present.

Antipruritics

Useful anti-pruritics for persistent itching include menthol (0·5%) or phenol 1% in aqueous cream, and calamine lotion, which contains arachis oil.

Barrier and protective preparations

These preparations protect against softening and maceration from moisture in flexures, for example the groins. They also have an occlusive effect. They are essentially bases with zinc oxide or silicone (as dimethicone). There are many preparations; some of the most commonly used are:

- Zinc cream BP, contains zinc oxide, arachis oil, and lanolin
- Zinc and castor oil ointment BP
- Conotrane (Yamanoouchi) and Siopel (Bioglan), contain dimeticone (dimethicone)
- Metanium (Roche), contains titanium dioxide
- Sudocrem (Forest) and Drapolene (Pfizer), contain lanolin.

Treatment for specific situations

Sunscreens

These give a degree of protection—mainly to ultraviolet B but also to ultraviolet A. They depend on their effect on a physical barrier (usually titanium dioxide) and chemicals that combine with epidermal cells, usually esters of PABA or oxybenzone.

Camouflage
Scars, congenital naevi and other blemishes that cannot be removed can be covered with suitable creams. Proprietary preparations are available.

Antiperspirants
Aluminium chloride for hyperhidrosis: aluminium chloride 20% (Driclor, Stiefel, or Anhydrol, Dermal Laboratories).

Depigmenting agents
2% hydroquinone cream is available without prescription as "fade-out". Preparations containing corticosteroids are also prescribed but not available as proprietary preparations.

Antimitotic agents
5-Flourouracil cream is useful for treating incipient malignancies—that is, solar keratoses, but not actual carcinomas. It is available as Efudix cream (Roche), which is applied daily for one to two weeks. It produces a variable degree of inflammation that is allowed to subside before the treatment is repeated.

Infestations
(1) *Scabies.* The correct procedure for treatment is more important than the preparation used. Benzyl benzoate 25% application BP is still available and is cheap but tends to irritate the skin. Malathion is available as Derbac (SSL), Prioderm (SSL), and Quellada M (Stafford-Miller), and Permethrin as Lyclear cream (Kestrel) preparations are more effective and less likely to irritate. 6% sulphur in white soft paraffin or permethrin are recommended for young children and pregnant or lactating women. The procedures for treatment set out on page 107 should be followed and clearly explained to the patient. For resistant cases ivermectin (Mectizan, MSD) by mouth is available on a named patient basis.

(2) *Pediculosis.* Preparations containing malathion, carbaryl, and permethrin are used either as shampoos or lotions. Lotions are most effective and should be left on the skin for 12 hours before washing off. The same preparations are available as for treating scabies, with the addition of 0·5% malathion lotion as Suleo-M (SSL). Recently a lotion of phenothrin (Full Marks, SSL) has become available for treating head and pubic lice.

Preparations for the mouth
Steroids—Adcortyl in Orabase (Squibb) or Corlan pellets (Evans). Both these preparations contain corticosteroids.

Antifungals—Daktarin (Janssen) or Fungilin lozenges (Squibb); Nystan (nystatin suspension, Squibb). Corsoidyl (chlorhexidine, GSK), and Difflam (3m Riker) are useful mouthwashes.

Topical immunosuppressants
Tacrolimus (Protopic, Fujisawa) has recently become available as an ointment in two strengths, 0.03% and 0.1%. It has not been evaluated in children under the age of two or in pregnant women. It is recommended that it is only used by dermatologists or those with considerable experience in treating eczema. Although the exact mode of action is unknown it does diminish T cell stimulation by Langerhan cells and diminishes the production of inflammatory mediators from mast cells. It should be used in moderate to severe atopic eczema that has not responded to either treatment. Skin irritation with burning, erythema, and pruritis are the most common side effects. In view of its immunosuppressive activity

any infection should be treated first and it should be used with caution if there is a risk of viral infection or if inoculations using attenuated or live organisms are being used.

Pimecrolimus (Elidel, Steeple Novartis) is a similar preparation recommended for intermittent treatment of eczema can also be used as an initial treatment for any flare up of eczema. It diminishes cytokine activity long term relieving both the erythema and pruritis of eczema.

In common with topical steroids any immunosuppressive drug should be used with caution as viral infections are likely to be present or the patient is undergoing inoculation with live or attenuated organisms.

Systemic treatment

Antibiotics are probably the most commonly used systemic treatment. Long term antibiotics are needed for acne and cellulitis. Antifungal and antiviral drugs are indicated if topical treatment is ineffective, particularly in the immunosuppressed, and when the infection has been confirmed by laboratory tests.

Immunosuppressant drugs have had a considerable impact on the treatment of autoimmune and connective tissue diseases and diminished the need for systemic steroids—previously the only treatment available. They are increasingly used for extensive and persistently inflamed dermatoses, particularly psoriasis and eczema.

Antibacterial drugs
All penicillins may cause allergic rashes, which may be severe, and the broad spectrum penicillins, amoxicillin, ampicillin, and co-amoxiclav, are particularly likely to cause an intense rash in patients with glandular fever. They tend to accumulate in patients with renal failure and may reduce the excretion of methotrexate which is used in the treatment of psoriasis.

Phenoxymethylpenicillin (penicillin V) is useful in Gram positive infections and erysipelas.

Flucloxacillin is used to treat infections due to penicillinase producing organisms. It is used in impetigo and cellulitis.

Amoxicillin and ampicillin are broad spectrum antibiotics but are destroyed by penicillinase. Co-amoxiclav is a combination of amoxacillin and clavullinic acid. It is effective against a wide range of organisms and beta lactamase producing staphylococci as well.

Cephalosporins are not affected by penicillinase and are effective against both Gram positive and Gram negative infections.

Ciprofloxacin is used for infections with both Gram positive and Gram negative organisms such as pseudomonas.

Erythromycin is used for the treatment of acne and is useful in Gram positive infections. Resistant strains of staphylococcus are appearing.

Metronidazole is useful for treating anaerobic infections and trichomonas infections. It is useful for rosacea that is not responding to conventional treatment.

Antifungal drugs
Topical treatment is usually effective but for fungal infection of the nails and intractable infections of the skin systemic treatment may be required.

Griseofulvin (500 mg daily) is a well established treatment for fungal infections of the skin, hair, and nails. Although it should not be used in pregnancy, it can be used in children. It can cause lupus erythematosus to flare up.

Terbinafine (250 mg daily) is an effective systemic antifungal drug that does not affect the liver. It is used for both nail and skin infections.

Imidazole and triazole drugs include itraconazole and ketoconazole, which are effective for dermatophyte infections of the skin and pityriasis versicolor.

Antiviral drugs

Discovery of drugs that inhibit viral DNA polymerase and inhibit their proliferation in vivo means that effective treatment for herpes simplex and zoster is now possible. They are effective at the early stages of infection and should be started as soon as symptoms appear. Aciclovir (Zovirax, GSK) is available as a cream.

Aciclovir is effective against both herpes simplex and zoster. The standard dose is 200 mg five times daily for five days. In varicella infections and herpes zoster 800 mg is given five times daily for seven days. It can also be given by intravenous infusion, and should be applied as soon as symptoms appear. In addition, it can be used for prophylaxis, particularly in the immunocompromised patients and atopics who are liable to fulminating infection.

Famciclovir and valaciclovir are similar and are recommended for treating herpes zoster.

Antihistamines

These drugs are used in urticaria and acute allergic (type I immediate hypersensitivity) reactions. The newer long acting and non-sedating antihistamines are useful for treatment during the day and can be combined with one of the sedating type at night if pruritus is preventing sleep.

Non-sedating antihistamines only cross the blood–brain barrier to a slight extent. They may cause arrhythmias, particularly terfenadine.

- Acrivastine (Semprex, GSK) 8 mg three times daily
- Cetirizine (Zirtek, UCB Pharma) 10 mg once daily
- Fexofenadine (Telfast, Hoechst) 120 or 180 mg once daily
- Loratadine (Clarityn, Schering-Plough) 10 mg once daily.

Sedating antihistamines

There are many available and which is used is largely a matter of personal preference. The sedating effect, which is enhanced by alcohol, means that they are best taken at night. They also potentiate CNS depressants and anticholinergic drugs. They tend to have anticholinergic effects, causing dry mouth, blurred vision, tachycardia, and urinary retention. Those commonly used are:

- Chlorphenamine (Piriton Stafford-Miller 4 mg daily)
- Cyproheptadine (Periactin (MSD) 4 mg up to four times daily)
- Hydroxyzine (Atarax (Pfizer) 10–25 mg at night; can be used during the day if drowsiness is not a problem)
- Promethazine (10 or 25 mg at night or twice daily)
- Trimeprazine (Vallergan (Castlemead) 10 mg two to three times daily).

Corticosteroids

In addition to topical preparations, systemic steroids may be required for the treatment of severe inflammatory skin conditions such as erythroderma developing from psoriasis or eczema. They are also used in vasculitis and erythema multiforme as well as connective tissue diseases. They are often required for the treatment of pemphigoid and pemphigus together with immunosuppressant drugs.

The side effects must be borne in mind, particularly for any long term treatment. Most important are given below.

Water and electrolytes
Sodium and water retention with loss of potassium.

Musculoskeletal
Osteoporosis, aseptic necrosis of the femoral head, growth retardation in children, and muscle wasting.

Ophthalmic effect
Cataract formation and increased tendency to glaucoma.

Other effects
Increase in blood pressure, peptic ulceration and fat redistribution, and impaired glucose intolerance.

Retinoids

These vitamin A derivatives have proved very effective in the treatment of psoriasis and acne but are not without risk of side effects. The most serious is that they are teratogenic and must be discontinued for at least three months after stopping treatment in the case of isotretinoin and five years after taking acitretin.

All patients should be warned of possible side effects and women of childbearing age must be using an effective form of contraception, which must have been used for at least a month before treatment has started as well as having a pregnancy test carried out. Liver function tests and fasting cholesterol and triglycerides should be carried out on all patients. After prolonged treatment in adolescence, radiological tests should be carried out to ensure that there is no extraosseous calcification. The most important side effects are:

- Abnormal liver function tests
- An increase in cholesterol and triglycerides
- Occasional increases in electron spin resonance and lowered white count.

Clinical side effects
Drying and roughening of the skin and mucous membranes, particularly the lips, can occur. There may also be thinning of the hair and nails. Photosensitivity eruptions can develop. Occasionally muscle and joint pains occur.

Acitretin
This drug is used for severe psoriasis including pustulosis of the hands and feet. It has also been used in other forms of keratosis such as Darier's disease and pityriasis rubra pilaris.

Isotretinoin
This drug is used for severe acne vulgaris that has not responded to antibiotics or other treatments. It is therefore often used in adolescence and it is important to be aware of the musculoskeletal effects and possible mood changes.

Immunosuppressants

Methotrexate
This drug is useful in severe psoriasis that is not responding to topical treatment. The main disadvantage is its adverse effect on the liver, which precludes its use in those who have alcoholic liver disease but who are often those most needing systemic treatments. Idiopathic immunosuppression can occur so a test dose must always be given and a full blood count carried out 48 hours later before treatment has started. There may be gastrointestinal upsets and osteometitis as well.

Methotrexate interacts with anti-inflammatory and antiepileptic drugs. A full list of drug interactions should be consulted before treatment is started.

After a 2·5 mg test dose and full blood count 48 hours later, the regular dose is 5–15 mg by mouth once a week. Full blood count and liver function tests should be carried out once a week for the first six weeks and thereafter once a month during treatment. Folinic acid should be given at the same time, as this prevents bone marrow depression. In many centres a liver biopsy is considered mandatory before treatment is started since blood tests will remain normal for some time during the development of hepatic fibrosis.

Azathioprine

This drug is used for systemic lupus erythematosus, pemphigus, and bullous pemphigoid. It enables the dosage of systemic steroids to be reduced. The most serious side effect is bone marrow suppression. This may occur quite rapidly, particularly in those with diminished ability to metabolise the drug. This is carried out by thiopurine methyl transferase (TMT). The level of this enzyme should therefore be determined before treatment is started and those at low levels given a lower dosage. Those who inherit high activity may require higher doses. Other side effects include gastrointestinal upset, liver toxicity, and an increased tendency to infection.

Ciclosporin

This drug has proved helpful in severe psoriasis within inflammatory lesions and, secondly, in the treatment of severe atopic dermatitis. There are a number of drug interactions and it is important to check renal function and monitor both blood urea and serum creatinine.

Other drugs

Dapsone

This drug was originally developed for treating leprosy but was proved very effective in dermatitis pityformis and some other conditions, such as pyoderma gangrenosum. It may cause haemolytic anaemia, and other side effects include bone marrow suppression, hepatitis, and peripheral neuropathy. Regular blood checks are essential.

Hydroxychloroquine

This drug is used in both systemic and discoid lupus erythematosus as well polymorphic light eruption and porphyria cutanea tarda. The most serious side effect is retinopathy but this does not occur if the dose does not exceed 6·5 mg/kg lean body weight.

Psoralens

These drugs are used in conjunction with long wavelength ultraviolet light as psoralen with ultraviolet A (PUVA) therapy described on page 67. It is used for the treatment of severe psoriasis. It has also proved effective in some cases of atopic eczema, T cell lymphoma of the skin, and occasionally in lichen planus. There is a risk of cataract formation, and a full blood count as well as antinuclear factor tests should be carried out.

Preparations for treating acne and varicose ulcers are described in the appropriate sections.

Further reading

Arndt KA. *Manual of dermatological therapeutics*, 5th ed. NewYork: Little, 1995

Appendix: Patient support groups

Acne Support Group	(0870) 870 2263
Behcet's Syndrome Society	(01488) 71116
Allergy UK	(020) 8303 8583
Cancer BACUP	(0808) 800 1234
British Association of Skin Camouflage	(01625) 267880
British Red Cross Skin Camouflage Service	(020) 7201 5172
British Leprosy Relief Association	(01206) 562286
Congenital Melanocytic Naevus Support Group	(0151) 281 9716
Darier's Disease Support Group	(01646) 695055
Dystrophic Epidermolysis Bullosa Research Association	(01344) 771971
Ectodermal Dysplasia Society	(01242) 261332
Ehlers–Danlos Support Group	(01252) 690940
Hairline International	(01564) 775281
Herpes Viruses Association	(020) 7609 9061
Ichthyosis Support Group	(020) 7461 0356
Latex Allergy Support Group	(07071) 225838
Lupus UK	(01708) 731251
Lymphoma Association (LA)	(0808) 808 5555
Marfan Association UK	(01252) 810472
Myositis Support Group	(023) 8044 9708
National Eczema Society	(0870) 241 3604
Neurofibromatosis Association	(020) 8547 1636
Pemphigus Vulgaris Network	(020) 8690 6462
Primary Immunodeficiency Association (PIA)	(010) 7976 7640
Pseudoxanthoma Elasticum (PXE) Support Group	(01628) 476687
Psoriatic Arthropathy Alliance	(01923) 672837
Psoriasis Association	(01604) 711129
Raynaud's and Scleroderma Association Trust	(01270) 872776
Scleroderma Society	(020) 8961 4912
Shingles Support Society	(020) 7607 9061
Telangiectasia Self Help Group	(01494) 528047
Tuberous Sclerosis Association	(01527) 871898
Vitiligo Society	(020) 7840 0855

Index

Page numbers printed in *italics* refer to boxed material

Index

Index

Index

Index

Index

vesicles 3
  in rashes 6
  see also blisters
viral infections 92–7
  AIDS-related 99
    see also HIV infection
  herpes viruses 92–3
  pox viruses 92, 93–4
  with rashes *95*, 95–7
  wart viruses 94–5
  see also individual viruses
virilising syndrome 54
vitamin A acid 49
vitamin D analogues 14
vitiligo 76, 84

warts, seborrhoeic 60
warts, viral 94–5
  AIDS patients 99
  treatment 95
    cryotherapy 115, 116

wen (sebaceous cyst) 64
wet soaks, eczema treatment 25
Whitfield's ointment 104
Wickham's striae *27*
Willi hair syndrome 55
"wrinkle lines," surgical excision 119
Wuchereria bancrofti 113

xanthomas 78, 79
  common types *79*

yeast infections 101, 103–4
  diagnosis and treatment 103–4, *104*
  see also candidiasis
yellow fever *105*
yellow nail syndrome 58

zinc oxide 26

140

The complete ABC series

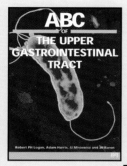

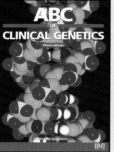

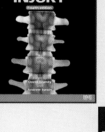

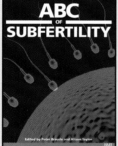

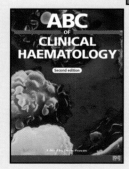

ABC of AIDS
ABC of Alcohol
ABC of Allergies
ABC of Antenatal Care
ABC of Antithrombotic Therapy
ABC of Asthma
ABC of Arterial and Venous Disease
ABC of Arterial and Venous Disease, CD ROM
ABC of Brain Stem Death
ABC of Breast Diseases
ABC of Child Abuse
ABC of Clinical Electrocardiography
ABC of Clinical Genetics
ABC of Clinical Haematology
ABC of Colorectal Cancer
ABC of Colorectal Diseases
ABC of Complementary Medicine
ABC of Dermatology (includes CD ROM)
ABC of Diabetes
ABC of Emergency Radiology
ABC of Eyes (includes CD ROM)
ABC of the First Year
ABC of Heart Failure
ABC of Hypertension
ABC of Intensive Care
ABC of Interventional Cardiology
ABC of Labour Care
ABC of Learning and Teaching in Medicine
ABC of Liver, Pancreas and Gall Bladder
ABC of Major Trauma
ABC of Mental Health
ABC of Nutrition
ABC of Occupational and Environmental Medicine
ABC of One to Seven
ABC of Oral Health
ABC of Otolaryngology
ABC of Palliative Care
ABC of Psychological Medicine
ABC of Resuscitation
ABC of Rheumatology
ABC of Sexual Health
ABC of Sexually Transmitted Infections
ABC of Spinal Cord Injury
ABC of Sports Medicine
ABC of Subfertility
ABC of Transfusion
ABC of the Upper Gastrointestinal Tract
ABC of Urology

Titles are available from all good medical bookshops or visit:
www.abc.bmjbooks.com